Wellbeing:
Policy and Practice

HEALTH AND SOCIAL CARE TITLES
AVAILABLE FROM LANTERN PUBLISHING LTD

ISBN	Title
9781908625144	A Handbook for Student Nurses, 2e
9781906052041	Clinical Skills for Student Nurses
9781906052065	Communication and Interpersonal Skills
9781906052027	Effective Management in Long-term Care Organisations
9781906052140	Essential Study Skills for Health and Social Care
9781906052171	First Health and Social Care
9781906052102	Fundamentals of Diagnostic Imaging
9781906052133	Fundamentals of Nursing Care
9781906052119	Improving Students' Motivation to Study
9781906052188	Interpersonal Skills for the People Professions
9781906052096	Neonatal Care
9781906052072	Numeracy, Clinical Calculations and Basic Statistics
9781906052164	Palliative Care
9781908625267	Pocket Guide for Radiotherapy
9781906052201	Professional Practice in Public Health
9781906052089	Safe & Clean Care
9781906052157	The Care and Wellbeing of Older People
9781906052225	The Care Process
9781906052218	Understanding and Helping People in Crisis
9781906052010	Understanding Research and Evidence-Based Practice
9781906052058	Values for Care Practice

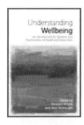

9781908625007

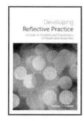

9781908625014

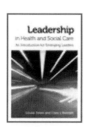

9781908625021

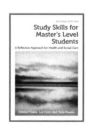

9781908625175

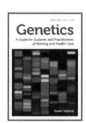

9781908625151

Wellbeing:
Policy and Practice

Edited by Anneyce Knight,
Vincent La Placa and Allan McNaught

Lantern

ISBN: 978 1 908625 22 9
Published in 2014 by Lantern Publishing Limited

Lantern Publishing Limited, The Old Hayloft, Vantage Business Park, Bloxham Rd, Banbury
OX16 9UX, UK

www.lanternpublishing.com

British Library Cataloguing in Publication Data
A catalogue record for this book is available from the British Library

The authors and publisher have made every attempt to ensure the content of this book is up to date and accurate. However, healthcare knowledge and information is changing all the time so the reader is advised to double-check any information in this text on drug usage, treatment procedures, the use of equipment, etc. to confirm that it complies with the latest safety recommendations, standards of practice and legislation, as well as local Trust policies and procedures. Students are advised to check with their tutor and/or mentor before carrying out any of the procedures in this textbook.

Typeset by Medlar Publishing Solutions Pvt Ltd, India
Cover design by Andrew Magee Design Ltd
Printed in the UK
Distributed by NBN International, 10 Thornbury Rd, Plymouth, PL6 7PP, UK

This book is dedicated to our children, friends and colleagues.

Anneyce Knight would especially like to dedicate this book to Bonnie Shirley Knight and the late Shirley Landels.

CONTENTS

ABBREVIATIONS AND ACRONYMS

ACPO	Association of Chief Police Officers
AIDS	Acquired Immune Deficiency Syndrome
BBC	British Broadcasting Corporation
BGS	British Geriatrics Society
BPS	British Pain Society
BRE	Building Research Establishment
CCG	Clinical Commissioning Group
CIEH	Chartered Institute of Environmental Health
CLP	Cultivating Lives Project
CPD	Continuing Professional Development
CQC	Care Quality Commission
DEFRA	Department for Environment, Food and Rural Affairs
DETR	Department for the Environment, Transport and the Regions
DH	Department of Health
EH	Environmental Health
EHRNet	United Kingdom Environmental Health Research Network
EOPIC	Engaging with Older People in Developing and Designing Interventions for the Management of Chronic Pain
EU	European Union
GCSE	General Certificate of Secondary Education
GDP	Gross Domestic Product
GP	General Practitioner
GYOC	Grow Your Own Club

HDI	Human Development Index
HEFCE	Higher Education Funding Council for England
HIV	Human Immunodeficiency Virus
HMO	Houses of Multiple Occupancy
HWB	Health and Wellbeing Board
IASP	International Association for the Study of Pain
IHDI	Islamic Human Development Index
JRF	Joseph Rowntree Foundation
JHWBS	Joint Health and Wellbeing Strategy
JSNA	Joint Strategic Needs Assessment
LA	Local Authority
LETB	Local Education and Training Board
LSOA	Lower Super Output Areas
LSP	Local Strategic Partnership
MENA	Middle East and North Africa
MMC	Muslim Majority Countries
MP	Member of Parliament
NEF	New Economics Foundation
NGO	Non-governmental Organisation
NHS	National Health Service
NICE	National Institute for Health and Care Excellence
ONS	Office for National Statistics
PARQ	Parental Acceptance Questionnaire
SECC	South East Coastal Communities
SEN	Special Educational Needs
SHS	Subjective Happiness Scale
SIG	Special Interest Group
SSM	Soft Systems Methodology
SWB	Subjective Wellbeing
U3A	University of the Third Age
UNDP	United Nations Development Programme
WHO	World Health Organization

THE CONTRIBUTORS

Allan McNaught has a background in health administration, health planning and development in the UK, transitional, lower and middle income countries, and as a university lecturer. He has previously taught at London South Bank, Greenwich and Keele Universities, as well as universities in Bosnia, Serbia and Zimbabwe. Currently he is an Associate Professor, and teaches hospital management and public health, at Hamdan bin Mohammed Smart University, located in Dubai in the United Arab Emirates (UAE). He is developing a research group to analyse the impact of the private health sector on health policy and health outcomes in the UAE. His main interest is in policy studies, particularly the role of social elites in the policy process, innovation in health care, and the international diffusion of health policy solutions.

Anneyce Knight worked in a number of roles within the NHS and the private sector before becoming a lecturer. She joined Southampton Solent University as Senior Lecturer in Health and Social Care in May 2013, from the University of Greenwich where she had held a number of roles. She led on the development of their BSc Health and Wellbeing and was European Lead and Erasmus Co-ordinator for the School of Health and Social Care. Anneyce is currently Course Lead on the innovative Joint Partnership Foundation Degree in Health and Social Care with Southampton NHS Foundation Trust and Health Education Wessex, which is integral to developing the new roles for Assistant Practitioners. She has published and presented on a variety of health and wellbeing issues, both nationally and internationally. She has also been a visiting lecturer at several international universities. Her research interests focus on Wellbeing (policy and practice) and Narrative Medicine, and she has a passion for the Health Humanities and their role in enhancing patient care.

Carlos J. Moreno-Leguizamon has a social sciences background in medical anthropology and health communication. He has extensive international experience, having worked in Colombia, the USA, India, Ghana, Tanzania, Kenya and the UK. Professionally, he combines two key areas of experience: on the one hand, programme design, implementation and evaluation of health, cultural and environmental projects and, on the other, teaching and researching health, culture and medical systems. In particular, his current research relates to the implementation of action research projects on Black Minority and Ethnic health issues in the South East of England. Carlos also teaches culture competency, compassionate care and equality and diversity at the University of Greenwich.

Christine Stacey has a nursing background and worked in a variety of clinical settings in the UK prior to spending sixteen years in the developing world where she circumnavigated the globe working with an NGO. Her interest and experience in working within international healthcare systems led her to the University of Greenwich as the Programme Leader for the BSc Nutritional Therapy. Her teaching interests lie with the emerging discipline of Psychoneuroimmunology and the socio-economic perspectives of health in both traditional environments and via e-learning. She teaches across the health and nursing programmes and is particularly interested in how student nurses learn in primary care placements and their understanding of the socio-economic determinants which impact on an individual's wellbeing.

David Smith is a Principal Lecturer in Sociology at the University of Greenwich. His research interests include social policy and welfare reform; the social impacts of economic change; social exclusion and the position of marginalised groups in contemporary societies. He is a member of the Gypsy Council and Gypsy Lore Society and has previously worked on projects related to the health, education and accommodation circumstances of Gypsy and Traveller communities. He has recently published a monograph *Gypsies and Travellers in Housing: The decline of nomadism* (2013, Policy Press) with Margaret Greenfields.

Jill Stewart's environmental health and housing career started in local government, leading to her current post as Senior Lecturer in the School of Health and Social Care at the University of Greenwich where she is a member of the Centre of Applied Social Research. She teaches across public health, housing and social work programmes to postgraduate level. Jill's main research interests include evidence-based practice and the effectiveness of front line strategies and interventions in sometimes very challenging public health and housing situations. She pioneered the development of the Chartered Institute of Environmental Health's Private Sector Housing Evidence Base. Her publications include books and numerous peer-reviewed articles in professional and academic journals and she has also presented papers at a range of conferences. She is currently involved in researching public health histories and is working with colleagues to explore novel methods of disseminating research. Jill was one of the founding members of the Environmental Health Research Network (EHRNet) which since its establishment in 2011 has delivered conferences, an ebook and website (at **http://ukehrnet.wordpress.com**).

Jim Gritton is originally a linguist by training. He enjoyed a successful career as a probation officer, rising to Assistant Chief Officer in the National Probation Service. After thirteen years in a variety of leadership roles, Jim embarked on a new career as a management consultant and co-founded a niche consultancy specialising in leadership and management development. He still undertakes occasional consulting assignments and has worked with a large number of public sector organisations, including central government departments, local authorities, emergency services, and the voluntary sector. Jim is currently Senior Lecturer in Leadership and Management in Health and Social Care at the University of Greenwich. Previously, he taught at the Open University (OU) Business School and continues to tutor on the OU's MBA programme. His main teaching specialisms are leadership, management and organisational behaviour, but he also teaches across several other academic disciplines, including public health, social work and criminal justice. He is a Fellow of the Institute of Leadership and Management and leads an international, interdisciplinary research project on experiential learning in virtual worlds.

Lynn Baxter has lived and worked in London for most of her life. She is a qualified primary school teacher, University Lecturer and Social Worker. She was a children and families Social Worker and Manager for 25 years. As a Child Care Coordinator and Independent Consultant, she developed particular interest and expertise in work with families with child welfare and protection concerns; domestic violence and in services to improve outcomes for Looked After Children. She has conducted research into parental participation in Child Protection conferences and she completed a study of young people, living in care, and their experiences of Review meetings. She has taught subjects related to her research to Social Workers and health and child care professionals, at the Universities of Sussex, East London and Greenwich and has also been an external examiner. She is the Chair of a Panel approving and reviewing Foster Carers for an independent Fostering Agency and is a member of the board of a theatre company specialising in social and forum theatre. She has two adult children, who also live and work in London.

Margaret Greenfields is Director of the Institute for Diversity Research, Inclusivity, Communities and Society (IDRICS) and a Reader in Social Policy at Buckinghamshire New University. Her research interests include ethnicity, poverty, gender and intersectionality. She has extensive experience of UK and international consultation, research and policy development on Gypsy, Traveller and Roma health and social inclusion issues. She also has interests and experience in diaspora/migration studies and faith-based social justice.

Maureen Rhoden is Senior Lecturer in the School of Architecture, Computing and Humanities at the University of Greenwich. She is a Fellow of the Chartered Institute of Housing and a member of the Association of Researchers in Construction Management. Maureen is also a member of the Research Group on the European Social Model (EUROsocial) Programme of the European Union, which is coordinated and funded by the International Foundation for Public Policies based in Madrid, Spain. Maureen has been an active researcher for the past twenty years and her primary interests are in Construction Management and the Built Environment.

Nevin Mehmet is currently the Programme Leader for the BSc (Hons) Health and Wellbeing at the University of Greenwich. As part of the Programme Leader role, Nevin is developing links within local health and wellbeing providers to support students with work experience in both statutory and non-statutory organisations. Nevin has a keen interest in community wellbeing and has undertaken several research projects that focus on this area. In addition, her previous role in providing holistic care within a primary setting has assisted in supporting and updating the BSc Health and Wellbeing, especially with regard to the health and wellbeing of individuals. Nevin has an MA in Medical Ethics and Law and teaches healthcare ethics to both undergraduates and postgraduates across the University's health and social care provision. Nevin's publications include chapters on 'Ethics and Wellbeing' in A. Knight and A. McNaught (Eds) *Understanding Wellbeing: An Introduction for Students and Practitioners of Health and Social Care* (Banbury: Lantern Publishing) and 'Legal and Ethical Aspects of Paramedic Practice' with Sam Willis, in S. Willis and R. Dalrymple (in press) *Fundamentals in Paramedic Practice* (Oxford: Wiley–Blackwell).

Pat Schofield currently works in the University of Greenwich leading the research agenda around pain, ageing and/or dementia. Professor Schofield has completed a number of funded post-doctoral projects around pain management in older adults and palliative care. She has also worked with groups of older adults providing them with research training, literature searching skills and developing service user-led research projects. Pat is currently involved in three major programmes of research around pain in older adults: a cross-council programme of research under the Lifelong Health and Wellbeing banner, entitled Engaging with Older People in Developing and Designing Interventions for the Management of Chronic Pain (EOPIC); a project on New Technologies to Support Older People at Home: Maximising Personal and Social Interaction, funded by dot.rural; and an EU-funded programme Pain Assessment in Patients with Impaired Cognition, especially Dementia. She has presented her work at a number of conferences in the UK and abroad and has many books and publications in the area. She is chair of the British Pain Society – Pain in Older Adults, Special Interest Group and chair of IASP Subcommittee on Education (Pain in Older Adults SIG) and is leading the BPS/BGS collaborative working group on pain.

Surindar Dhesi is a chartered environmental health practitioner and is completing a PhD at the University of Manchester, which is exploring how the new English Health and Wellbeing Boards are approaching the task of tackling health inequalities, with particular reference to environmental health. Her research interests also include public health, local government, evidence-based practice and health policy. She is a founder member of the UK Environmental Health Research Network (EHRNet), which aims to develop a research and publications profile in the environmental health profession. Surindar is also a guest lecturer on Communicable Disease and Environmental Health at Oxford Brookes University. As an environmental health practitioner, Surindar is Director of Gage Health & Safety Limited which specialises in providing environmental health support for large event organisers and caterers. Prior to this she worked for ten years in local government environmental health, most recently as Health and Safety Team Leader at Birmingham City Council, on secondment to the Health and Safety Executive as the Midlands Partnership Liaison Officer. Surindar wishes to acknowledge, with thanks, the contribution of Dr Anna Coleman, who kindly commented on a draft of Chapter 4.

Vincent La Placa is Senior Lecturer in Public Health and Policy at the University of Greenwich where he specialises in public health, sociological theory and quantitative and qualitative research methodologies. Prior to that, he worked as a Research Consultant at the Department of Health, where he managed the qualitative phase of the Healthy Foundations Life-stage Segmentation. Vincent's PhD focused on the social and psychological construction of sexual and familial relations and identities among gays and lesbians and their immediate families, using quantitative and qualitative methodologies. He has presented at national and international conferences and published numerous reports and papers on a variety of theoretical and empirical research, including post-positivist research in health policy and the emergence of social tourism and leisure policy within organised modes of capitalism. His most recent activities have focused on the discursive emergence of wellbeing in public health discourse and the impact of modern capitalism on policy development and intervention strategies.

01

INTRODUCTION

Anneyce Knight, Vincent La Placa
and Allan McNaught

THE CONCEPT OF WELLBEING

The concept of wellbeing is currently being explored globally and underpins some policy areas within the United Kingdom (UK). Governments and policy makers are debating how to use and measure wellbeing, beyond the traditional means that focus singularly upon material and economic indicators. This book seeks to develop the contemporary research evidence base for health and wellbeing within a global context and focuses on the changing perspectives on health and wellbeing. It is written by a multidisciplinary group who have extensive national and international experience across the statutory and non-statutory sectors. It presents the many different but interconnected arguments around wellbeing and its relevance to modern societies and communities.

UK Government policy is increasingly placing health and wellbeing at the centre of public policy. Health and wellbeing is conceptualised in a holistic manner, to include, for example, individual, psychological, social and environmental (and even spiritual) elements. An example of this is the announcement in 2009 by the National Institute for Health and Care Excellence (NICE), that schools should 'measure' the 'happiness' and wellbeing of children in the classroom. Wellbeing, it is argued, is affected by, for instance, negative parenting and familial relationships. Negative parenting and poor quality family or school relationships place children at risk of, for example, poor mental health. This recognition is also part of a broader shift from a focus on parent and child 'relations' to the 'quality' and effects of the 'couple / family' relationship upon child outcomes (Bingham, 2013). At the same time, the UK public health structure is witnessing historic alterations, such as the incorporation of concepts of choice, consumerism and evidence-based medicine in intervention development and healthcare services, and organisational restructuring of healthcare systems. This can be seen in the form of devolvement of local responsibility for healthcare and the emergence of Health and Wellbeing Boards to account for and ameliorate the health of local populations. La Placa and Knight (2014) argue that this affords public health professionals the opportunities to develop locally based concepts of wellbeing, engage communities in its development, and create links to debates around social capital acquisition and the influence of structural determinants; for instance, poverty and social exclusion. In terms of healthcare delivery, La Placa and Knight (2014) also argue that recent changes call for collaboration between local statutory and voluntary organisations in applying locally produced concepts of wellbeing to public health policy, and engaging with healthcare interventions, grounded within local context and needs (La Placa *et al.*, 2013a; La Placa and Knight, 2014).

There has also been increasing recognition that successful outcomes of policies cannot be judged only by the effects of economic or material indicators, but that a more contextual and qualitative assessment, among others, is often required. For example, the Treasury is now required to add wellbeing in any appraisal of policy, as are other Departments throughout Whitehall. Moreover, the Office for National Statistics (ONS) has devised an official index to measure the nation's 'happiness'. The shift towards wellbeing in government policy requires a focus upon how we define and measure the concept, how it can be incorporated into policies and outcomes, and unpack its relations with concepts, such as 'health' and 'illness'. It requires that we look at it from a theoretical and practical perspective, if the concept is to be developed throughout Whitehall, and made meaningful to policy makers, professionals and lay people alike. Currently, there is no concrete agreement around what constitutes wellbeing, its relationship with other policy discourses around, for example, poverty and education, or the most effective means of measuring impact and designing policy interventions. This book seeks to address theoretical perspectives whilst presenting practical examples of policy discourse and intervention development in health and wellbeing research. It intends to add to the developing body of evidence to contribute to enhancing the knowledge base around the delivery of the health and wellbeing agenda, both in terms of policy and practice.

Global economic turbulence also lends weight to the contention that policy makers and practitioners need to develop new ways of measuring and assessing wellbeing beyond material and economic indicators, as well as defining its relationships with concepts of health and disease. The globalisation of healthcare and lifestyles, witnessed in late modern societies, also acts as an incentive for policy makers and practitioners to discuss complexities and changes in health and wellbeing policy and practice.

THE AIMS AND CONTENT OF THIS BOOK

This book focuses on wellbeing broadly in policy and practice and proceeds to look at it in different contexts. It seeks to incorporate and integrate the broader aspects of wellbeing within the national and global policy context, as opposed to traditional discourses. These tend to view wellbeing solely as a measurable psychological or economic phenomenon, often separate from broader socio-economic and environmental concerns. The intention is to make current debates and policies accessible to a wide audience in the research, practice and policy making communities, and seeks to precipitate debates around how they can collaborate to maximise the concept of wellbeing in their work. Health and social care workers and policy makers, local authority employees, the public health community, wellbeing and social care practitioners and students will find the book particularly helpful and engaging in dealing with theoretical concepts and practical issues.

Book chapters are contained within two parts. Part One deals with Wellbeing: Policy and Practice, and Part Two with Wellbeing: Contextualised. Part One contains three chapters, dealing with theoretical and policy issues. Carlos Moreno-Leguizamon, in Chapter 2, problematises the concept of wellbeing in the health and social care sciences and the potential challenges assumed as a result. In Chapter 3, Vincent La Placa and Anneyce Knight chart the late modern emergence and 'breaking in' of wellbeing as a new policy phenomenon, both globally and in the UK, paying particular attention to the role of global neo-liberal ideology and Thatcherism that opened up spaces for its development and revision. The chapter also considers how the impacts of these shifts affect theory, policy and research around wellbeing. It argues that public policy should shift attention to how individuals and social groups construct wellbeing through a plurality of discourses, articulation of needs and competing cultural and material exchanges, resources, and economic contexts, reflecting changes in the national and global context. In Chapter 4, Surindar Dhesi discusses the role of Health and Wellbeing Boards in current UK policies and the impact upon health inequalities and environmental wellbeing.

Part Two contains six chapters, dealing with wellbeing in practice and its uses, and proceeds to view wellbeing as a tool for interventions and measurement of outcomes in an increasingly diverse policy environment, served by various policy communities. In Chapter 5, Jill Stewart and Jim Gritton examine the relation between wellbeing and housing and the way this contributes to debates around promotion of wellbeing in the living environment.

In Chapter 6, David Smith and Margaret Greenfields draw attention to wellbeing for Gypsies and Travellers, employing the concept of 'cultural trauma' to explain the adverse collective outcomes of rapid and sudden changes in traditional lifestyles and contexts faced by gypsies and travellers. In addition, the chapter considers how forms of cultural resilience and resistance to assimilation can mitigate the more traumatic aspects of settlement and enhance individual and collective wellbeing for group members. In Chapter 7, Anneyce Knight, Vincent La Placa and Patricia Schofield consider the implications of wellbeing on older people, particularly the relationship between neo-liberalism, Thatcherite policies in the UK and elderly care, and they examine some of the issues for older people that this presents. Ways in which these issues are being tackled are further explored in the chapter. Anneyce Knight, Jill Stewart, Maureen Rhoden, Nevin Mehmet and Lynn Baxter use Chapter 8 to explore the implications for wellbeing by providing a case study of a seaside town, affected by declining tourism and a local economy, and the partnership model used to enhance family and community wellbeing, in the light of decline, and the challenges presented. In Chapter 9, Nevin Mehmet and Christine Stacey explore the proliferation of garden schemes and urban beautification which can enhance wellbeing. The chapter examines the underpinning theory and practice that support such initiatives and discusses the current research that supports expansion of these types of schemes to promote holistic wellbeing. In Chapter 10, Allan McNaught proceeds to advance a global perspective, and explores policy, definitions and the assessment of the wellbeing of Muslim populations in the Middle East, North Africa and South East Asia. He further explores the influence of culture and religion, and compares and contrasts the Islamic view with Western concepts of wellbeing.

Finally, in the conclusion which forms Chapter 11, Anneyce Knight, Vincent La Placa and Allan McNaught attempt to draw together the existing theoretical and policy discourse, and research and evidence knowledge base. They contend that wellbeing has emerged as a discursive late modern phenomenon, the uniqueness of which lies in the development of modern capitalism, and that enables it to be articulated and used in modern policy discourse, and within less traditional contexts. However, the challenge lies in the abilities of policy makers and healthcare professionals to design policies and interventions that make wellbeing seem 'real' and 'relevant' to the population, as a whole. Wellbeing must be made to 'mean' and 'feel' something among lay people, and be perceived to be relevant to policy and public health outcomes among professionals. Wellbeing should be a two-way relationship between lay populations and professionals. It needs grounding in a 'double hermeneutics' (Giddens, 1993), understood by all communities, if it is not to be passed off as a 'fad' or abandoned by future governments. The individualisation of self and society carries the risk that wellbeing interventions revert solely to individual psychological interventions. However, new means of theorising concepts of wellbeing lend greater weight to its development and reduce the risk that it might one day be forgotten.

Another challenge lies in policy makers' and healthcare practitioners' ability to generate discourses and interventions, in a world where traditional methods and ways of viewing 'wellbeing', 'satisfaction' and 'happiness', for instance, have changed dramatically, but where current forms and modes of capitalism have remained largely unchanged, despite recent austerity and fluxes in modern economic systems. Such debates present further challenges towards, for example, choices between local and generic wellbeing interventions and the relationships between different and competing segments of the UK population. The globalisation of culture and economies may also witness a shift to global definitions of wellbeing, adding another complex, but rich, discourse to the policy making process and establishing wellbeing as a core concept in the twenty-first century. We hope we have begun this process.

PART ONE
WELLBEING: POLICY AND PRACTICE

02

WELLBEING IN ECONOMICS, PSYCHOLOGY AND HEALTH SCIENCES: A CONTESTED CATEGORY

Carlos J. Moreno-Leguizamon

"And yet at stake in this struggle over the corpse of epistemology are some of the most important spiritual issues of our time".

(Taylor, 1989: 485)

AIMS OF CHAPTER:

- To identify the contemporary construction of the idea or category of wellbeing as discursively constructed from the social sciences; in particular, economics, psychology and health sciences;

- To promote reflection upon the central value of this idea or category, not only for the conduct of research from a social sciences perspective, but also for new social policies.

INTRODUCTION

This chapter aims to present a comprehensive and critical overview of the contemporary, emergent, conceptual category of wellbeing as it is being constructed by various social science discourses; in particular, economics, psychology, and health sciences. Broadly defined, wellbeing is an ever-changing category that, at least in the West, emerged within Greek philosophy, particularly Plato's and Aristotle's characterisation of happiness as that desirable state of virtue implicitly comprising a norm that encapsulates a value judgment about one's life (Mehmet, 2011). This value judgment also includes the meaning of living life in positive terms, namely 'a good life'. Another element related to this definition is the dominance of the positive effect over the negative effect, i.e. the prevalence of pleasant emotions over unpleasant ones (Bourne, 2010; Cameron *et al.*, 2006; Diener, 2009a; McNaught, 2011; Moreno-Leguizamon and Spigner, 2011; Spigner and Moreno-Leguizamon, 2011). In view of its history, and the contemporary reinterpretations to which it is being subjected, wellbeing is a category that the economic, psychological and health sciences discourses are attempting to grasp mainly by 'scientifically' quantifying variables, scales, indexes or synonyms such as quality of life, life satisfaction, subjective wellbeing and even happiness itself from a positivist epistemology.

Thus, this chapter, in order to survey critically the prevailing construction, production, and circulation of the category of wellbeing within these three discourses, addresses two interrelated and overlapping points. First, the chapter reviews and discusses from an epistemological angle (the positivist angle) the main definition of wellbeing and all its synonyms – happiness, quality of life, life satisfaction and subjective wellbeing as used currently by the various discourses – in order to observe similarities and contrasts among the conceptualisations. Secondly, the chapter attempts to suggest some alternatives to the common positivist conceptualisation of wellbeing by discussing three very relevant issues around the wellbeing category: *Is this a relative or a universal category?*; *Is it a subjective or objective category?*; *Is it a category of meaning that is context dependent or context independent?* The emphasis on the epistemological angle – how we know what we do about wellbeing – is significant in unpacking how the category is produced and circulated to a lesser degree, thus creating the most prominent challenges and limitations. The chapter closes with some suggestions to be taken into account in the definition of this category from an ontological perspective based on Castoriadis' work, as discussed by Tovar-Restrepo (2012) and Tomlinson (1991).

It is anticipated that the chapter will contribute to a richer debate on wellbeing from a social sciences framework, as well from as a trans-disciplinary perspective for different audiences. First, for the academic audience (health practitioners, psychologists, social scientists and economists) the chapter will demonstrate the debate over constructing and reproducing a category – in this case wellbeing – from a single epistemological angle (the positivist one), which is the one predominantly used in mainstream economic, psychological and health sciences discourses. Secondly, for policy makers the chapter will illustrate what it means, contemporarily, to construct the category of wellbeing as a parallel to income and growth, concepts that have been, in their own right, powerful notions that give a sense of reality, identity and power to societies and governments.

Happiness, quality of life, subjective wellbeing, life satisfaction and wellbeing

An overall glance at the production and circulation of the category of wellbeing and all its synonyms demonstrates that, despite an exhaustive amount of methodological and theoretical effort over the last fifty years (Diener, 2009a; Diener, 2009b; Diener and Diener, 1995; Diener et al., 1995; Diener and Seligman, 2002; Diener et al., 2003; Graham, 2011; Nussbaum and Sen, 2006), the mainstream economic and psychological discourses and, to a certain extent, the health sciences discourses concentrate primarily on the quantification of wellbeing from a positivist epistemology. In other words, some of the basic positivist assumptions underpinning the construction, production and circulation of the category of wellbeing are as follows:

- Neutral valuation or objectivity constitutes a mediating value when ascertaining the facts explaining wellbeing;
- Since the natural sciences and social sciences are assumed to be one (methodological monism), wellbeing can be an 'object', measurable, predictable and controllable, based on a cause–effect model and production of general laws (Alderson, 1998; Jones-Devitt and Smith, 2007; Moreno-Leguizamon and Spigner, 2009);
- This category, regardless of complexity, multidisciplinarity and multidimensionality (Bourne, 2010), can be measured and, therefore, known through increasingly sophisticated tools, surveys and scales, empirical research and 'hard data' (Alderson, 1998);
- This category is primarily orderly, systematised and knowable through indicators such as quality of life and life satisfaction at either the individual level or the social level.

Thus wellbeing was useful in providing some of the first comprehensive, global measures of wellbeing across the individual, family, community and social domains but simultaneously excluded the richness of this category from other epistemologies, such as the phenomenological, the social-constructionist or the post-structuralist, to name but a few. Hence, there are some common interesting observations to be made as a result.

Happiness

Firstly, although the literature reviewed in the three disciplines insists on characterising happiness as the most open-ended, general and ambiguous of all the categories, this is the most 'sexy', catchy and widespread of all when it comes to its use in titles of books and academic articles. As mentioned earlier, its basic definition goes back mainly to the conceptualisation of a good life and all the virtues as discussed by Aristotle (Mehmet, 2011). Economists, however, also include in the characterisation of happiness Jeremy Bentham's concept of hedonic utility which, according to Graham (2011), means the maximisation of contentment and pleasure to the greatest number of people as they go through the experience of living. That happiness can be measured objectively, as assumed by positivism, is a common assumption in the three discourses. For instance, a source in economics states that "The economics of happiness approach provides us with new tools and data with which to develop measures of welfare that include income metrics but also extend well beyond those metrics" (Graham, 2011: 7).

Quality of life

Secondly, quality of life, the next synonym of the category of wellbeing, is, like happiness, used interchangeably in the three discourses, although it means something slightly different from wellbeing as such and within each discipline. In general, quality of life, as Mathews and Izquierdo (2009) state, means external observations and evaluation by people of their level of satisfaction with external conditions rather than their internal states of mind or psychological factors, as pointed out by Bourne (2010). Similarly, in one of the classic works on quality of life in economics, Nussbaum and Sen (2006: 1), in a very revealing epistemological sentence, state that "we need, perhaps above all, to know how people are enabled by the society in question to imagine, to wonder, to feel emotions such as love and gratitude that presuppose that life is more than a set of commercial relations…". The paradox here is that, despite Nussbaum and Sen's significant effort to enrich the discussion of quality of life from a philosophical point of view in this seminal work, the psychological and health sciences discourse in general and the economic discourse in particular continue to insist on a quantitative language made out of scales and indices such as the Physical Quality of Life Index or the Happy Planet Index, which will provide an optimal measure. Meanwhile, in contrast to the economic discourse in health sciences, the category of quality of life has a meaning more related to the individual and the impact that life has naturally (age) or accidentally (becoming disabled) on him or her. And, like the scales that are expected to measure quality of life in societies collectively, the scales used in health sciences are expected to measure individual quality of life.

What seems to have been forgotten in all these exercises in measuring and designing scales and indices is what Griffin (2002) ironically says about any quantitative language, namely, that it is only able to construct reality between the 'more' and the 'less'. Griffin (2002: 75) states: "There are many scales of measurement, and it would be astonishing if wellbeing were not measurable on at least one of the less demanding ones". Thus, the fact that quality of life can be measured objectively as an external situation, if it is disaggregated in more narrow components, such as life expectancy, education, health and so forth, is also a positivist assumption here. And although the meaning in economic and health sciences discourses varies, since the first one emphasises the external environment and the second one focuses on the individual, the emphasis of both is on objectivity and measurement. Additionally, of the three discourses, the one that speaks less about quality of life is the psychological one. In this discourse, the synonymous category to emphasise, when attempting to explain wellbeing, is life satisfaction.

Life satisfaction

Thirdly, life satisfaction is the next interchangeable synonym characterising the category of wellbeing and is mainly produced within a positivist epistemology. The influence of the psychological discourse on this category is significant since its basic meaning derives from the feelings and emotions of how people feel about their lives in various dimensions: time (past, present and future) interpersonal relations (social aspects) and the self (self-esteem, self-perception and self-concept). Furthermore, Graham (2011) adds two attributes to this category: income and assessment of people's lives from a whole perspective rather than an immediate one, as happiness does. Moreover, when inquiring about life satisfaction, the classical methodological question is encapsulated in the statement about people's level of satisfaction with their lives. The issue in terms of the production of this category from an epistemological perspective is that it is associated with the objective measurement of economic growth or prosperity in terms of national and individual incomes (Moreno-Leguizamon and Spigner, 2011) on the one hand and, on the other, the search for scales that enable us to infer people's level of satisfaction with their lives. What is very particular about the use of this category, in terms of the three discourses, is the influence of the basic definition of the psychological discourse on the health and economic discourses in compelling them to include emotions and feelings. As we know, the disciplines of mainstream economic and health sciences discourses are not comfortable with handling emotions as most of their assumptions are based on the behaviour only of rational individuals.

Subjective wellbeing

Fourthly, the next definition used interchangeably with the category of wellbeing, also from a mainly positivist epistemology, is subjective wellbeing. According to Graham (2011) and Diener (2009a), it encompasses all the ways in which people report their wellbeing: that is to say, from a person's belief in his or her life as something desirable, pleasant and good, in an open-ended way, to satisfaction with different domains such as work, health and education, and even life itself. The classical and most extensive work on the conceptualisation of this category is that by Diener *et al.* (1995). For reasons of space, this chapter is unable to describe this work in detail. However, the most general trait of this extensive and pioneering work, from an epistemological dimension, is the contemporary re-appropriation of the old philosophical notion of happiness, albeit this time made 'scientific' through its operationalisation by supporting experimental and empirical research. The wide-ranging work on measuring subjective wellbeing, through the operationalisation of all types of variables and scales, situations and life events, without giving any consideration to incommensurability and subjectivity of the researcher, is perhaps the most notable trait. The presumption that psychological discourse, as well as economic discourse, is a science fits very well with Putnam's (2006) criticism of the separation of facts and values: "[Y]et even today, economists whose philosophical ancestry is logical empiricism still write as if the old positivist fact / value dichotomy were beyond challenge" (ibid., 2006: 144). Thus, the critical element in this definition from the epistemological angle is whether subjective wellbeing pertains just to an individual and his or her feelings, or whether an individual and his or her feelings are in constant enactment with others and in the socio-economic, cultural and political environment in which the individual lives.

Wellbeing

Fifthly, we come to the definition of wellbeing itself, as used by the three mainstream discourses, and the one encompassing all the synonyms discussed above. The main trait, as pointed out earlier in another article (Moreno-Leguizamon and Spigner, 2011), is that its meaning derives from two very pervasive streams in contemporary discussion: first, the subjective and objective aspects involved in the definition of the category of wellbeing and all its synonyms; and, secondly, the differences in the production, circulation and distribution of the category by the three discourses.

The first aspect, the subjective and objective elements in the discussion of wellbeing and its synonyms, can be regarded mainly in two ways: on the one hand, the subjective aspects of what is experienced as a good life in terms of the internal feelings and emotions of the individual (the very good influence of the psychological discourse); and, on the other hand, what constitutes a good life as an external situation experienced by the individual in terms of objective conditions, i.e. what any collectivity such as society, culture, government, group or family provides to him or her, including the issue of rights (economic and, to a certain extent, health science discourses). The various definitions illustrated above demonstrate this.

Defining the category of wellbeing itself, the New Economics Foundation sees the category as incorporating "two personal dimensions and a social context: life satisfaction, people's personal development and people's social well-being" (Moreno-Leguizamon and Spigner, 2011: 59). Lastly, another definition that attempts to be more comprehensive on the matter of subjective and objective comes from the UK Department for Environment, Food and Rural Affairs (DEFRA); it states that it is "a positive physical, social and mental state: it is not just the absence of pain, discomfort and incapacity. It requires that basic needs are met, that individuals have a sense of purpose, that they feel able to achieve important personal goals and participate in society" (DEFRA, 2009).

With respect to the differences in the production, circulation and distribution of the category of wellbeing and its synonyms by the three discourses, the differences and similarities are as follows. For example, in the health sciences discourse, what is defined as wellbeing displays an internal debate and tension between biomedical sciences and social sciences, since it is considered that this category is still firmly based on the biomedical definition of health, in contrast to bio-psychosocial (emotions and feelings), environmental, socio-economic and political definitions of health (Bourne, 2010; Moreno-Leguizamon and Spigner, 2011; La Placa *et al.*, 2013a). The paradox here, as also pointed out earlier, is that this occurs despite the progressive efforts by the World Health Organization to define health, in 1948, as not merely the absence of disease in the restricted biomedical sense of the term, in order to include wellbeing. Hence, the dominance of the biomedical definition of health and, therefore, wellbeing methodologically translates to the common use of quantitative language in health sciences based on the very basic assumptions of positivism. Be it health or wellbeing, the issue is to develop scales, indices and units that can measure these phenomena objectively.

There are only marginal efforts in fields such as public health or community health, to think of health and wellbeing as more qualitative phenomena and thus view them from other epistemological angles such as the phenomenological, post-modernist or post-structuralist (Cameron *et al.*, 2006; Moreno-Leguizamon and Spigner, 2009).

Meanwhile, in the psychological discourse, the definition of the category of wellbeing is chiefly subjective wellbeing as discussed above, denoting the individual's experience and whether he or she feels that life is something desirable, pleasant and good (Diener, 2009a). Although this is significant for bringing the emotions and feelings to the debate, elements that have been lacking in the so-called 'rational' economic and health sciences discourses, the methodological production and circulation of this category comes from a positivist angle. In this search for an objective category, the psychological discourse attaches itself firmly to facts emerging from empirical research, something that Diener (2009b) considers mainly as the methods of science.

In the case of the economic discourse, the category of wellbeing has so far been translated, to a certain extent, into quality of life; moreover, like the psychological discourse, it is assumed that it can be constructed as a 'scientific' category through the use of experimental or empirical research with the addition of a political dimension, such as a discussion of quality of life within a human rights frame. A significant peculiarity in the construction of wellbeing, and the other synonyms for the economic discourse, is the global financial crisis that began in 2007 and, in particular, the search by some governments for alternative notions to income and growth that earlier offered legitimacy to both economic discourses and key performance indicators of governments but are now revealing signs of exhaustion. The reductionism and bias with which the notions of income and growth have been produced and circulated cannot be ignored here. Governments in different parts of the world are currently asking economists to develop an index of wellbeing that runs parallel to such dubious notions as income and growth. Fortunately, some of them are incorporating what the psychological discourse is saying in terms of emotion and feeling, in contrast to the merely 'rational' subject, which has been the bread and butter of that discipline. Historically, income and growth have been at the core of measuring and, hence, classifying the level or ranking of development or wellbeing of a society without an adequate understanding of what wellbeing might mean or represent for the various groups that comprise any society in terms of ethnicity, gender, disability, sexual orientation, age and religion. Thus, it seems paradoxical that wellbeing is now being accorded significance against the backdrop of a global financial crisis. Ultimately, this is why it is necessary to understand how this category will be multidimensional, trans-disciplinary, multifaceted but incomplete if treated only from a positivist angle.

BEYOND THE POSITIVIST DEFINITION OF WELLBEING

Since the 20th century, the search for alternatives to a positivist way of knowing and its assumptions from other epistemological angles has been varied. For example, from the phenomenological, social constructionist and post-structuralist discourses, albeit with different accents, there have been some serious criticisms of the golden rule of objectivity as a value when coming to know, produce and circulate a category like that of wellbeing. Similarly these discourses consider that human beings, rather than explaining what they know (as in positivism), make inter-subjective and subjective interpretations – sense making – of their reality.

Another challenge to the positivist way of knowing is the all-pervasive obsession with treating the methodology of the natural sciences and the social sciences as one, thereby creating the dominance of quantitative language, which becomes trapped in the circular argument of the 'more', 'equal' or 'less', as pointed out earlier by Griffin (2002). For example, in a very interesting critique of the overemphasis on the mathematisation of the economic discourse, and probably the psychological and health sciences discourses, via empirical research, Sedlacek (2011) states that "we have overemphasised the mathematical and neglected our humanity. This has led to the evolution of lopsided, artificial models that are often of little use when it comes to understanding reality. I argue that mainstream economists have forsaken many colors of economics, which ignores issues of good and evil. We have created a self-inflicted blindness, a blindness to the most important driving forces of human action" (ibid: 8). Also at stake here is the issue of incommensurability, which is nothing less than the careful consideration that not everything is comparable, and that, if it is, it requires serious contemplation. Despite the importance and significance of the quantitative angle, the point to add is that the knowing of human beings, let alone their wellbeing, is not exhausted by quantitative methods.

Another issue of interest for those angles contesting the assumptions of the positivist way of knowing comes from the critique of the overemphasis on the rational human being and his or her truth as implied by the mainstream economic, psychological and health sciences discourses. For those angles wishing to go beyond positivism, again with important variations, the possibilities of the human being are not exhausted by the rational, and the truth is relative. This opens up the debate on whether the meaning of wellbeing is relative or universal, a subjective or objective or a context dependent or context independent category.

From very innovative approaches (Bok, 2010; Thin, 2009; Tovar-Restrepo, 2012; Tomlinson, 1991), some brief answers can eventually be elucidated. For Bok (2010), the exploration of happiness as a category has to be related to philosophy, religion, art, literature and narrative (the subjectivity side of human beings). Meanwhile, for Thin (2009), from an anthropological and ethnographical angle, the universal, equally important to the relative, should come from three suggested assumptions: feeling well is important for most people in most places; most cultures differentiate between 'feeling well' and 'living a good life'; and people's moral codes are oriented towards helping others to feel and live well, except in certain situations (i.e. punishment, lack of democracy, authoritarianism and so forth).

Lastly, from an angle more ontological (ontology of creation) than epistemological – based on the work of Cornelius Castoriadis – Tovar-Restrepo (2012) and Tomlinson (1991) introduce the concept of the imaginary signification of society to observe that, for that thinker, this concept informs the real and the rational, and, from here, the need to go beyond these values to recover our critical thinking ability. "An imaginary signification is a representation which is neither 'real' in the sense of being available to perception and empirical scrutiny nor 'rational' in the sense of being deducible via the rules of thought of a culture. But this does not mean it is either unreal or irrational in the pejorative sense that these terms possess in modern Western culture…it is the product of an act of [social] creation which is fundamental to any subsequent system of cultural representation" (Castoriadis, cited in Tovar-Restrepo, 2012: 156–7). For Tovar-Restrepo, the value of thoughts such as those of Castoriadis comes from "his elaborations on the individual and social poles of the subject [which] throws light on the old problem in the social sciences of whether the subject should be considered an individual agency or a collective product, and the false belief that society is the sum of individual subjectivities" (Tovar-Restrepo, 2012: 136). The subject as an undetermined entity is equipped with radical imagination and therefore a creative one, self-mediated by social institutions, even those that attempt to define what is, or should be, her or his wellbeing.

CONCLUSION

This chapter aimed to discuss critically and problematise the contemporary construction of the category of wellbeing and all its synonyms (happiness, quality of life, subjective wellbeing, life satisfaction and wellbeing) as defined and used by social science discourses, especially economic, psychological and health sciences discourses. Examining what those discourses are, or are not saying about wellbeing, the chapter attempted to reconstruct this category from the positivist epistemological angle rather than the methodological or theoretical angles from which numerous research studies have been produced and circulated.

It has been assumed that it is from the epistemological angle that the category of wellbeing eventually displays most of the innovative, multidimensional, trans-disciplinary and multifaceted aspects that are not always as harmonic, complete or consensual as the positivist epistemology suggests. The lack of production and circulation of the category of wellbeing from distinct epistemological angles such as the phenomenological, social constructionist and post-structuralist ones (to name but a few), has prompted economic, psychological and health sciences discourses and, in particular, the ontology of creation to point out the lack of clarity, the rather incomplete nature, and the complexity of a conceptual category such as wellbeing. And this is something that economic, psychological and health sciences discourses should recognise when these discourses assume the power and authority to design policies and prescribe meaning.

RESEARCH POINTER 2.1

According to the main discussion of this chapter on the production and circulation of the category of wellbeing and all its synonyms (happiness, quality of life, subjective wellbeing, life satisfaction and wellbeing), select at least five abstracts from the literature on each discipline (economics, psychology and health sciences) in which this topic is being discussed.

Keeping in mind mainly the positivist assumptions presented in this chapter, try to respond to the following questions:

- Does the article mention the use of any theory related to wellbeing?

- What is the main methodological approach of the article (quantitative, qualitative or both)?

- Does the article refer to particular scales, indices, surveys or questionnaires related specifically to the measuring of wellbeing?

- Is there any argument related to the subjectivity and self-reflection of the researchers reporting their research findings on wellbeing?

FURTHER READING

Bok, S. (2010) *Exploring Happiness: from Aristotle to brain science*. New Haven, CT and London: Yale University Press.

Mathews, G. and Izquierdo, C. (2009) *Pursuits of Happiness: well-being in anthropological perspective*. New York: Berghahn Books.

Tovar-Restrepo, M. (2012) *Castoriadis, Foucault, and Autonomy: new approaches to subjectivity, society and social change*. London: Bloomsbury.

03

WELLBEING: A NEW POLICY PHENOMENON?

Vincent La Placa and Anneyce Knight

AIMS OF CHAPTER:

- To consider the emergence of wellbeing as a new policy phenomenon in public health and the processes that have given rise to it;

- To locate wellbeing within the global and national context;

- To focus upon potential ways of studying and analysing the concept of wellbeing in public health as a result of the conditions that have shaped its emergence.

INTRODUCTION

The concept of wellbeing has emerged as a new paradigm within current UK government policy discourse and recent changes to the public health structure. The origins of wellbeing as a central concept in public health are linked to the development of late modern capitalism and pluralism that has witnessed it 'breaking' in to UK public health policy discourse (La Placa and Knight, 2014). Additionally, it is connected to the global and national policy context that has also seen significant changes over the last thirty years. This chapter outlines these developments and the processes that have shaped wellbeing as a new policy phenomenon. It argues that given recent changes, public policy should shift attention to how individuals and social groups construct wellbeing through a plurality of discourses, articulation of needs and competing cultural and material contexts and resources. Wellbeing, as a guide to policy development and outcomes assessment, should be intrinsic to UK government policy and public health practice, reflecting continued social change and individuals' ability to construct and negotiate their wellbeing, security, and quality of life.

WELLBEING AND CONTEMPORARY POLICY IN THE UK

Debates around concepts of wellbeing or happiness were initially precipitated within the philosophy of ethics, particularly morality and how one could use it to judge how 'satisfying' or 'conformist' one's life was in terms of decisions made (Mehmet, 2011). Sociologists have approached it from the individual perspective, whereby individuals subjectively constructed ideas around wellness or wellbeing, often with regard to the effects of wider objective social structures and communities on interpretations (La Placa *et al.*, 2013a). Contemporary debates around wellbeing have also produced an increasing array of literature and policy discourse (McNaught, 2011) that often problematises concepts of wellbeing since initial references were made to it by the World Health Organization (WHO) in 1946, which said that "health is not the mere absence of diseases but a state of wellbeing" (WHO, 1946). These debates have focused on the complex and contingent nature and domains of wellbeing as much as the relationship between individual subjectivity and wider determinants in articulating it. As such, the concept of wellbeing is nebulous and contested (Knight and McNaught, 2011). It often requires analyses within both local and broader contexts, as well as how individuals and communities construe and apply it, either to individual decisions and choices and/or large-scale policy discourse and development.

The debate has assumed significance in public health policies since 2010, where the government's approach has been to view wellbeing as a strategic priority, an outcomes tool, and a new and distinct paradigm in policy discourse (La Placa *et al.*, 2013a). In 2010, the UK government made a commitment to measure and assess 'individual' and 'psychological' wellbeing, using indicators such as 'satisfaction', 'anxiety' and 'happiness' (La Placa *et al.*, 2013a). The emergence of wellbeing in public health policy discourse had also witnessed multiple definitions throughout policy initiatives under the Labour administration between 1997 and 2010. The Department for Environment, Food and Rural Affairs (DEFRA) (2009) defined wellbeing as meeting 'individual' need, giving sense of 'purpose' in terms of 'personal relations', financial reward' and 'attractive environments'. The Department of Health's (DH) (2009) consultation document, *New Horizons: towards a shared vision for mental health*, defined wellbeing as a positive state of mind and body, ability to feel safe and cope with a sense of connection with people, communities and the wider environment.

Building upon this, policy makers have increasingly conceptualised wellbeing, not only in traditional terms of absence of pain and disease, but how it is produced through individual action and its policy impact for wider communities (Department of Health, 2010a; 2010b). It often views health and wellbeing as one and the same, produced on the social, physical, psychological and environmental level, suggesting that wellbeing is a multi-levelled definition, even if it is not comprehensively articulated as such. However, undoubtedly, there appears to be a new emphasis upon the individual's ability to negotiate and articulate what promotes wellbeing in interaction with wider domains, particularly local communities. Clearly, there is much scope for defining and articulating wellbeing in public health as a result.

Changes to the public health system in the UK over the past decade have also embedded concepts of wellbeing within national policy discourse and healthcare structures. For example, the government is encouraging a focus upon meeting the needs of individual and community wellbeing by transferring public health and policy decision-making to local government. It is also encouraging local communities to devise and implement health and wellbeing strategies and interventions, aligned to local needs (Humphries *et al.*, 2012). The establishment of local Health and Wellbeing Boards, for instance, will conjoin commissioning of local NHS services, social care and health improvement strategies through consultation and partnership with local communities (Humphries *et al.*, 2012). They will also assume responsibility for advancing health and wellbeing improvement and prevention activity. A core function is to formulate a Joint Strategic Needs Assessment (JSNA) and this will be used to agree combined local action in the form of a Joint Health and Wellbeing Strategy (JHWS). The Health and Social Care Act (2012) has also ensured that the JSNAs have authority to inform local commissioning decisions by the Clinical Commissioning Groups, Local Authorities and the NHS Commissioning Board. The aim is to encourage local constructions of wellbeing, affording local communities opportunities to define needs and respond to them through local public health infrastructure and resources. The chapter now proceeds to focus on the broad historic and discursive emergence of wellbeing as a new phenomenon in public health policy and discourse.

THE EMERGENCE OF WELLBEING AS A NEW POLICY PHENOMENON

The emergence of wellbeing as a central concept in public health is linked to a historical and discursive process that has seen it 'breaking in' to UK public health policy discourse as a discrete idea in its own right and as a new public policy concern, as opposed to traditional ones around welfare and economic growth (Bochel, 2009). It is a late 20th and early 21st century discourse that has been produced through the broad emergence of modernity (be that late or post-modernity) that now characterises the West, at least. Other new and emerging concerns have been, for example, wellbeing at work, leisure, quality of life and environmental sustainability (Bochel, 2009). However, it has also been influenced through the national UK political context that has sought to respond to wider global social and economic change and frame policies within a specifically national context.

From the Second World War onwards, wellbeing, if articulated at all, was used mostly within the context of economic growth, materialism, and enhanced levels of income and Gross Domestic Product (GDP) and its effects on an individual's prosperity (Kavanagh, 1990). Wellbeing was an economic and individual concept with a focus on individual materialism and how the economy could consistently enhance this. Development of the economy, and continued enhancement of living standards, were perceived as the core ethical concept in ensuring happiness and advancement of wellbeing. Keynesian demand management, full employment and economic inclusion were the paramount precepts in ensuring an increasing higher standard of living and therefore enhanced wellbeing for all classes (Kavanagh, 1990). Linked to this was the belief in expertise (Kavanagh, 1990), that expert knowledge and direct government intervention could manage both capitalist modes of production and social policy to enhance continued growth and consequently wellbeing. This was often accompanied by the belief that a society organised around collective structures, universal policies and bureaucracies, was best served by positivist modes of inquiry, knowledge and policy (Comte, 1975).

The social world was viewed as empirical and the discovery of invariant societal laws and relations would lead the way to the progressive and universal organisation of society and the economy. Once this was in progress, it was believed that this would be reflected in enhanced satisfaction with both economic and personal wellbeing and happiness. Neither was wellbeing (if acknowledged at all) defined or conceptualised as a specific framework for policy within its own right, but usually classified as one domain within a limited biomedical discourse around physiological health and absence of pain and disease. Health, like concepts of bureaucracy and economic organisation, was best captured and improved through the lens of universal empiricism and narrow biomedical concepts of, for example, pain and physiology (La Placa et al., 2013a). Social and health science sought to understand the totality of human action and relations, restricting it to empirical observation and universal explanations which would advance happiness and economic wellbeing. Both the physical and social worlds could be controlled for the betterment and enhanced satisfaction of society.

However, the development of late modern societies in the late 20th and early 21st centuries has created space to develop and refine concepts of, for instance, bureaucracy, economics, and consequently wellbeing, and its place within public health. As modern capitalism, consumerism and new forms of knowledge and relationships advance, individuals and communities become less reliant on traditional and previously arranged patterns of thought (Giddens, 1990; 1991). Individuals have more choice to develop and revise previous actions and local modes of thinking as modern capitalism has evolved up to the present day. Individuals find themselves confronted by new and less traditional relationships, identities and situations where traditional early and mid-20th century responses are no longer as relevant. As a result, the concept of 'radical reflexivity' emerges (Giddens, 1990; 1991). This means individuals consistently re-examine all aspects of their lives and relations, responding to new ways of constructing the 'self' and negotiating new relations and situations outside tradition-bound contexts.

Traditional and established forms of thought erode and individuals become more aware of a plethora of information systems and choices in seeing to their needs. Linked to this is the demise of class and socio-economic status as significant determinants of individuals' identities and life-course, as individuals construct their own biographies and lifestyles more fluidly (Giddens, 1990; 1991). The self is no longer embedded in traditional and institutional groups or class-bound relationships that define how one behaves or defines pre-determined needs. Rather through the 'reflexive project' of the self, individuals are freer to define and determine their own needs and lifestyles.

The consequence of this is that individuals and communities are faced with new and enhanced issues around, for example, 'trust' and 'risk'. Modernity generates a distinctive risk profile as a result of the large-scale change it brings about as regards economics, society and radical reflexivity. Risk also becomes global in intensity as individuals experience the growth of contingent events that affect large numbers of people across the globe. Recognition of these risks increases a sense of insecurity and the need to think about and readjust need, security enhancement and happiness. Individuals search for a greater sense of trust and connection with themselves and the external world to achieve 'ontological security' (Giddens, 1990; 1991). The search for trust, stability and security is predicated upon recognition that what occurs on a global level has immense influence upon how we construct our personal needs, identities and sense of self (Beck, 1992). Hence, social and public policy evolves to represent and enable solutions to problems that traditional concepts of social policy no longer provide answers to. The breaking in of the concept of wellbeing in modern policy discourse is one aspect of this and seeks to provide policy and intervention solutions relevant to late modern capitalist societies.

Greater choice, renewed interest in concepts of lifestyle, consumerism, risk, and developments in global technologies, used to shape and define concepts of global and individual security and need, enable lay individuals, healthcare practitioners and public health policy makers to revise previous 'traditional' concepts of wellbeing that narrowed happiness and satisfaction to economic circumstances or physiology. Wellbeing is a broader and contested concept that focuses on happiness, quality of life, security and need, and how individuals and groups respond to ever-changing circumstances that cannot be addressed by traditional empirical economism alone (although clearly the economic domain of health and wellbeing remains important). This provides space to construct and give meaning to the multiple domains that affect both public health and wellbeing and give consideration to the greater influence and impact of these on policy and practice. For example, McNaught (2011) argues for wellbeing as a broad policy concept that goes beyond traditional views of health as disease focused, to the wider determinants of, for example, families, neighbourhoods and communities, and how individuals utilise the resources available within them. Not only does this approach maintain the links between public health and wellbeing, but it perceives promotion and enhancement of wellbeing as a collective effort (national and local) and not just a matter of individual psychology or economics.

Habermas (1990; 1992) also argues that the greater complexity and differentiation that characterise current capitalist societies have brought about many benefits in terms of, for example, science and technology. For instance, new knowledge around health, disease and lifestyle enables individuals to live healthily and survive diseases that would have ended their lives in the early 20th century. Nevertheless, he also surmises that whilst rational thought systems and technological changes can facilitate security and healthier lives, they can also precipitate insecurity and lack of trust in individuals' subjective 'life-worlds' as they construct complex biographies and relationships that are constantly in flux. This can prevent individuals and communities from flourishing and creating the happiness and satisfaction in their personal lives that they perceive as relevant to wellbeing.

Habermas (1990; 1992) suggests that the solution to this would be to devise a society which appreciates the social, physical and psychological impact upon people and how anxiety and insecurity might be mitigated as a result (McNaught, 2011). An emergence of an effective civil society in the form of, for instance, voluntary organisations, social movements or interest groups, can vocalise causes in the hope that the public sphere and government might respond and take action. Civil society enables enhanced equality, social justice and critical thinking around how best to attend to the needs of individuals, as well as the production of new and competing discourses within which to frame these strategies, often referred to as 'communicative action' (Habermas, 1990; 1992). Clearly, the concept of wellbeing, and its place in achieving this type of society, will have a central place in developing social and public policy around individual, community and global requirements. This is what Habermas (1990; 1992) refers to as the 'unfinished project' of modernity, the wellbeing of social systems on the structural and individual levels. Wellbeing is a reflexive form of analysis that can harmonise both levels and produce effective results for individuals. It is a new concept to provide solutions where traditional ones can no longer be relied upon to enhance happiness, stability and security.

Others argue that modern capitalist societies are best referred to as 'postmodern' societies (for example, Lyotard, 1984; Peters and Marshall, 1996). 'Postmodernity' transcends late modernity and is subject to more rupture and change than suggested by those who subscribe to late modernity. Under the postmodern condition, grand truths and singular narratives cannot capture the complexity of the modern world or the required public and social policy responses. Concepts of progress, scientific knowledge, lifestyles and wellbeing are in constant flux and can only exist within the current discourses and policies that articulate them. This is predicated on the belief that there can be no singular articulation of wellbeing, wellbeing policies, and interventions that would not eventually descend into a singular and totalising strategy. Emphasis is on a plurality of definitions and power relations that construct them. Any attempt at defining wellbeing objectively or economically automatically ignores the multiple social and cultural power relations that bring these definitions into existence. There is no unity as to the development of ideas or policies in the policy making process. Rather, one analyses how the different parts of the policy making process approach an issue. For example, what are the reasons for the lack of consensus around definitions of wellbeing by the state and whose interests do multiple definitions serve?

The emergence of wellbeing specifically on the UK policy agenda, and in current modern policy discourses, also requires analysis of the national context as well as most recent global developments. The national context in the UK has largely mirrored events and developments across the West since the end of the Second World War. Faith in planned economies and government intervention to iron out inequality through the welfare state has been replaced by neo-liberal ideology (Stedman Jones, 2012). Neo-liberalism espouses free markets, individualism, consumerism and the belief that social engineering by state intervention is detrimental to economic and social freedom and should be discouraged (Ferguson *et al.*, 2002).

NEO-LIBERALISM, THATCHERISM AND WELLBEING

The dominance of neo-liberal ideology since 1979 has had a mixed impact upon the definition and location of wellbeing on the policy agenda. In the 1980s, wellbeing was never articulated or developed explicitly as part of the Thatcherite agenda. If it was acknowledged at all, it was in the guise of how free markets, freedom to choose, competition and individualism increased choice and prosperity and therefore enhanced individual wellbeing. Nevertheless, it is inappropriate to reduce Thatcherism (however one defines it) to the realm of classical economics only. Letwin (1992) and Saunders (2012) argue that Thatcherism was as much a moral, ideological and discursive project as it was about economic transformation. One can argue that it had the capacity to change and redefine discourses and events beyond economics. For example, the moral and 'virtuous' emphasis upon 'individual choice' and 'freedom to choose' were eventually reclaimed and applied to personal and moral issues around, for example, personal relationships and sexual wellbeing. If economic wellbeing could be enhanced through markets, freedom to purchase, and diversity of choice, why could the same not apply to, for instance, family, sexual and other relationships? Why could freedom to choose in the material marketplace, not translate into freedom to choose in other areas of identity and personal life? The values of economic liberalism and commercialism extended into areas that deepened the need to think more about wellbeing, quality of relations and individual and community needs, beyond the economic realm.

For example, the increase in lesbian and gay visibility (both socially and commercially) and the greater acceptance of sexual diversity and freedom in the 1980s as a result, gave rise to issues around sexual rights and sexual health and wellbeing; particularly the wellbeing of those with HIV/AIDS (often translated into political AIDS activism). The entrance of more women into, and the diversification of the labour market brought changes in how we perceived, for example, the rights and wellbeing of women in the family and the workplace. New articulations of child wellbeing were also evident in the Children Act of 1989 that reflected increased choice in familial relations, and recognised changes in childhood experiences due to diversity in parenting and family structure. Thatcherism significantly widened the scope of wellbeing beyond classical economics and introduced new modes of thought that enabled individuals and new social movements to define their needs and wellbeing. This was often achieved through harnessing new technological developments, such as the internet, to promote their interests on the policy agenda (Bochel, 2009).

Early 21st century changes to the public health structure and agenda in terms of emphasis upon, for instance, localism, choice, diversity of service, and articulation of individual and community need, can also trace their origins back to developments in the 1980s and thereafter. Furthermore, despite the dominance of neo-liberal ideology, the UK has largely remained wedded to an 'organised' form of modern capitalism (Habermas, 1992). This is where government continues to assume significant responsibility for social and economic wellbeing in terms of the welfare state and public expenditure, despite the priority given to and reliance upon free markets and individualism.

As a result, the UK has had, and continues to have an active civil society, which is independent of the economic sphere and can challenge current modes of thinking around neo-liberalism, relationships and wellbeing. As Chanan and Miller (2013) argue, the presence of social movements, campaigning organisations and community groups continues to pressure national and local government in the UK for better services, enhanced social rights and services conducive to wellbeing. 'Empowerment' and 'involvement' are integrated with 'delivery of services', 'community action' and 'participation' (Chanan and Miller, 2013). The increase in community practice, neighbourhood renewal, area-based initiatives to reduce poverty and discourses around 'the duty to include' and 'engage with local and voluntary communities' is further evidence that civil society has the capability to define and promote issues around wellbeing (personal and social) within hegemonic neo-liberal discourse.

POLICY AND PRACTICE: WELLBEING, CULTURES AND INDIVIDUALS

The decline of traditional economics and positivist methods of empiricism that accompanies the emergence of late modern societies is important for wellbeing policy and practice. Horkheimer and Adorno (1972) argue that a scientific method of social science stifles and devalues human knowledge, emotion and sensibilities if they are perceived to be subject to control and prediction. Through such methods, populations are eventually targeted and controlled by the state in its interest (Horkheimer and Adorno, 1972). Rather, the emergence of pluralism and individuals' ability to manage time and space, interpret their surroundings, and challenge traditional modes of thinking, has the potential to enable 'self-actualisation' and the capacity to negotiate with and alter systems of regulation and control.

The concept of wellbeing is intrinsic to self-actualisation, encompassing a plurality of public health and wellbeing issues that affect our lives from, for instance, sexual practices, management of emotions, resilience, positive psychology, mechanisms for coping with personal and social change, through to traditional public health concerns, such as smoking, drinking and body weight. This is not to deny the role of experts and professionals in constructing and organising potential systems of guidance and regulation, but to realise the potential of people to articulate and renew conceptions of health and wellbeing in a world of greater choice and flux (Dalmayr, 1986). Wellbeing has emerged through a particular historical process of late modernity, but will be articulated and sustained through further processes that renew and re-contest it, both on the individual and structural levels.

Jordan (2008) suggests an appropriate response to wellbeing policy development, given the decline of empiricism and the traditional economic model of assessing wellbeing and/or happiness. He suggests analyses of the forms of activities and exchanges that transform human and material resources into personally and socially valued goods through interpretation and negotiation. Much of this occurs within different organisational and cultural institutions throughout civil society that transcend consumption and economics. Interactions produce and distribute symbolic social value influenced through cultural practice and bond individuals together. Cultural transformation is intrinsically bound up with wellbeing. Definitions of wellbeing, and policies around how societies produce and promote it, are bound up with multiple collective and cultural institutions and exchanges, as much as with economic exchange (Jordan, 2008).

Wellbeing is contingent upon how individuals relate to one another and how this is constructed and understood within cultures. Policy can enable and direct such activity, but it is less likely to be able to determine it through planning or prediction (Jordan, 2008). The study of how wellbeing is influenced through such interaction should become the central focus for policies directed at happiness, quality of life, life worlds and self-actualisation. Individuals and social groups become the core concern. Focus can shift to how they compete for resources and compare their requirements to those of others. Policy can provide for collective solutions where possible, but can recognise increased complexity and differentiation in forms of exchange and competition for resources and security. As such, policy makers and practitioners are required to rethink traditional responses of, for instance, wealth redistribution and/or planning for need and focus upon new and varied responses. This is also bound up with late modernity's turn towards choice, change and pluralistic response to social and material change.

Changes to the UK public health structure in terms of decentralisation and local delivery of services provide, we believe, a basis to encourage this policy response, enabling individuals and local communities to develop meaningful and local concepts of wellbeing, whilst considering local social determinants such as the physical environment, income, and the implications for public health practice. Definitions of wellbeing and subsequent policies can transcend traditional economistic and biomedical views, enabling individuals and communities to engage and define specifically local and culturally bound constructs of wellbeing. New ways of thinking about and applying wellbeing afford opportunities to challenge attempts at constructing singular and hegemonic definitions, be they economic or physiological. This shifts public policy attention to the competing needs of different groups, which will inevitably be different, and which change in response to people's ability to reflexively alter their circumstances.

Neither does this strategy assume that consumer capitalism in its late modern form (or indeed neo-liberalism) is necessarily detrimental to wellbeing or self-actualisation as argued by critical commentators of social policy (e.g. Ferguson *et al.*, 2002). As we have argued previously, wellbeing is historically contingent upon both the development of late modern capitalism and national neo-liberal responses to it. Yet the new modes of thinking, encouraged by late modernity, also have the potential to develop discourses of wellbeing that can be integrated into or challenge neo-liberalism directly. An example of this is the incorporation of concepts of wellbeing and happiness in the emergence of 'social tourism' (tourism and leisure as a tool for social inclusion, social capital acquisition, and enablement of positive social relationships); and its challenge to commercial tourism (as a mechanism for the development of tourism purely for commercial purposes, profit and material relationships) (La Placa and Corlyon, 2013).

CONCLUSION

This chapter argues that the concept of wellbeing has emerged as a historical and discursive construct linked to the development of late modern capitalist society. It is an alternative to traditional biomedical views of health and economistic means of defining and assessing happiness and satisfaction. It is also grounded within new forms of exchange, relationships and social changes. Public policy should shift attention to how individuals and social groups construct wellbeing through a plurality of discourses, articulation of needs and competing cultural and material exchanges, resources and economic contexts. The shift to decentralisation and local delivery of health and wellbeing services in the UK should encourage this process further. Concepts of wellbeing in all its forms, as a guide to policy development and outcomes assessment, should be intrinsic to UK government policy and public health practice, reflecting continued social change and individuals' ability to construct and negotiate their wellbeing, security and quality of life.

RESEARCH POINTER 2.1

Think about how your parents and grandparents might have perceived their own wellbeing and how this is, if at all, different when compared with what wellbeing is to you?

- Now list potential reasons why this might be and some appropriate policy responses.

FURTHER READING

La Placa, V., McNaught, A. and Knight, A. (2013) Discourse on wellbeing in research and practice. *International Journal of Wellbeing*, 3(1): 116–125.

Walker, P. and Marie, J. (2011) *From Public Health to Wellbeing: the new driver for policy and action*. Basingstoke: Palgrave.

Bok, D. (2010) *The Politics of Happiness: what government can learn from the new research on well-being*. New Jersey: Princeton University Press.

04

THE ROLE OF HEALTH AND WELLBEING BOARDS

Surindar Dhesi

AIMS OF CHAPTER:

- To describe the background, development and work of the new English Health and Wellbeing Boards;

- To consider their role in addressing health inequalities which impact on local health and wellbeing;

- To refer to findings from an empirical research project which explored how Health and Wellbeing Boards are tackling health inequalities, with a focus on the role of environmental health.

INTRODUCTION

Health and Wellbeing Boards (HWBs) are new English structures which went 'live' in April 2013, and are essentially a unique form of 'upper-tier' or unitary local authority (LA) committee. Their uniqueness relates to their statutory membership, which includes council officers, elected members, representatives from General Practitioner Clinical Commissioning Groups (CCGs) and others, all of whom have equal voting rights. The HWB structure provides the first occasion on which all the statutorily listed members are legally required to work together to improve local health and wellbeing; a specific duty to encourage integrated working between health and social care set out within the Health and Social Care Act 2012. They are also expected to prioritise tackling health inequalities (Peate, 2012; The Association of Directors of Children's Services *et al.*, 2011).

This chapter includes data from a doctoral research project (Dhesi, 2014) which used qualitative research methods (semi-structured interviews, observations of meetings and analysis of HWB documents) at four longitudinal case study sites in the Midlands and north of England. In addition, semi-structured interviews were carried out with Environmental

Health (EH) practitioners and managers from all English regions. In total, 50 interviews took place and 23 HWB meetings were observed. Data were collected over a period of eighteen months, including the 'shadow' and early 'live' phases of HWB development, and were thematically analysed using ATLAS.ti.

HEALTH AND WELLBEING BOARDS

The idea and introduction of HWBs were generally welcomed and seen as the least controversial part of the changes to the health and public health systems in England under the Health and Social Care Act 2012, although there were some who dismissed claims that they would improve the democratic legitimacy of the NHS (Fitzpatrick, 2011).

Statutory members of HWBs include council officers (Directors of Adults' and Children's Services and Director of Public Health), an elected member (usually the Council leader or portfolio holder for health), CCG representatives, and a member of the local Healthwatch. These are new organisations representing patients and the public. A representative of NHS England must also attend when the Joint Strategic Needs Assessment (JSNA) and Joint Health and Wellbeing Strategy (JHWBS) are discussed and, if requested, when their commissioning functions are discussed (Department of Health, 2012a).

Many HWBs have also included non-statutory members; for example, additional elected members, representatives of lower-tier authorities (i.e. district and borough councils), the police, healthcare providers, the voluntary sector and other organisations. Non-statutory members have equal voting rights with statutory members and the number of HWB members in each area is variable, ranging from fewer than twelve to more than twenty (Humphries *et al.*, 2012). Very few HWBs have environmental health directly represented.

HWBs are required to meet in public and this doctoral research, with its focus on HWBs, health inequalities and environmental health, has found that these Boards often have in excess of twenty observers, usually from the local health economy, attending meetings. In some areas, these observers are permitted to contribute to the meeting or are asked for their views or present papers, whilst in others there is little interaction with HWB members until the end of the meeting.

The Department of Health describes HWBs' functions as

> "...bring[ing] together those who buy services across the NHS, public health, social care and children's services, elected representatives and representatives from HealthWatch to plan the right services for their area. They will look at all health and care needs together, rather than creating artificial divisions between services." (Department of Health, 2011).

Interestingly, whilst there are many references to health, social care and 'health related services' there is no definition or explanation of 'wellbeing' in the legislation relating to HWBs.

HWBs are required to carry out a JSNA, followed by a JHWBS to meet the identified needs of the local population. CCGs and LAs will be required to commission 'in line with the health and wellbeing strategy' (Behan, 2011: 2; Pulse, 2011) and this will 'encourage a shared understanding of local priorities' (Behan, 2011: 1). Since they do not have statutory powers, HWBs rely primarily on political (and other) leadership and influences (Humphries *et al.*, 2012; Sillett, 2012). They do not have any real powers to enforce change, cannot apply sanctions, and cannot veto commissioning plans (Calkin and Ford, 2011); this has been described as a 'soft' role (Staite and Miller, 2011: 9). An example of this HWB soft role is the 'power to encourage close working (in relation to wider determinants of health)' (Department of Health, 2012b: 3). It is difficult to envisage how this power 'to encourage' could effect real change in areas where parties are reluctant to cooperate or leadership is weak. *Figure 4.1* shows the theoretical route of HWB influence on local commissioning decisions.

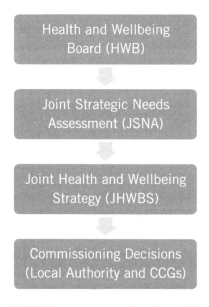

Figure 4.1 *The theoretical route of HWB influence on commissioning decisions.*

My research on HWBS, health inequalities and environmental health has found HWB member involvement in preparing the JSNA and JHWBS to be variable; in some areas they have been drafted primarily by the team of the Director of Public Health, with limited involvement of HWB members, whilst in other areas, members have been fully involved in the process. Some have called for HWB members to conduct an audit of their JSNA and to ensure that it is 'owned' by parties outside public health (Harding and Kane, 2011). It was found that the preparation of these documents in the first year was often in the form of a 'refresh' of the existing JSNA and strategies, which is a practical solution, given the early stage of HWB development and tight timescales involved. The preparation of JSNAs has been required of upper-tier LAs and the NHS since 2007, so they are not new. However, the responsibility of the multi-agency HWB to produce a strategy is novel (2011). Somewhat strangely, whilst the HWB must prepare the JSNA and JHWBS, it does not have a duty to publish them, as this responsibility lies with the CCGs and LA (Department of Health, 2012b).

The promotion of joint working between professional groups in health and social care is also not new and has been the focus of many former policies and strategies, although the majority of these initiatives have met with mixed or limited success and it is thought that HWBs 'are likely to face similar challenges' (Humphries *et al.*, 2012: 8). Others have voiced concerns that the ability of the new commissioning system to make an impact will be limited by financial pressures and a loss of skills and expertise during the restructuring of services (Turner *et al.*, 2013). However, government expectations around the ability of HWBs to deliver have been high since the idea was first mooted (Behan, 2011; Sillett, 2012).

HEALTH INEQUALITIES

Health inequalities are complex and enduring and have been called 'wicked problems' (Hunter *et al.*, 2010: 158). It is widely accepted that there are links between mortality rates and age, gender, class and employment (Mitchell *et al.*, 2000) and that with some exceptions, poorer people are associated with shorter lives and poorer health and wellbeing than richer people (Benzeval *et al.*, 1995; Davey Smith, 2003). This is known as the 'health gradient', meaning that between and within every social class, 'the higher the position, the better the health' (Marmot and Wilkinson, 2006). It is also known that advantaged groups are also experiencing faster health gains than less advantaged groups (Graham, 2009). There is a great deal of evidence to support the existence of health inequalities between social groups and in different geographical areas; for example, there is a north/south divide in England, with people in the more affluent south living longer, illustrated by the 9.2 year life expectancy difference for males in East Dorset and Blackpool (ONS, 2013). These statistics describe a great deal of avoidable pain, suffering and lost years. As Marmot says, 'Inequalities are a matter of life and death, health and sickness, well-being and misery' (Marmot *et al.*, 2010: 37).

Curiously, there is no consensus definition of what health inequalities are and it is therefore unsurprising that the term will mean different things to different people. This research has found this to be the case at some HWBs, where although there is enthusiasm to find consensus, there were differences in the perceptions of health inequalities of some interviewees, which was reflected in the discussions around prioritisation for action.

There are very many explanations offered for why health inequalities exist and Bartley (2004) helpfully describes four different models: behavioural and cultural; psycho-social; materialist; and life-course approaches, covering a wide range of theories ranging from poor housing to cumulative life events. (Readers with a deeper interest in these models will find Bartley's book listed in the 'Further Reading' section below).

Other theories include the idea that the prolonged stress of a 'social-evaluative threat' creates a constant 'fight or flight' reaction, where cortisol is released, leading to physical effects including cardiovascular problems and obesity, and psychological effects such as increased aggression (Wilkinson and Pickett, 2010). An alternative theory proposed by Scott-Samuel is that health inequalities stem from societal power inequalities. These include the neo-liberal capitalist system (Coburn, 2004), the lack of emotional literacy in leaders and the patriarchal religious system which he says will prevent any progress being made in the current context (Scott-Samuel, 2011). There are also many other theories relating to specific groups such as women, ethnic minorities and people living in certain geographical areas. In measuring these (and the traditional class) factors, there have been criticisms of the lack of information and routine recording of information required to measure health inequalities (Fulton, 2010; Townsend *et al.*, 1988).

The 'life-course' approach was subscribed to by Marmot *et al.* (2010) in their strategic review of health inequalities and subsequently adopted by the government (Department of Health, 2010b). This explanation of health inequalities began with the work of Forsdahl and later Barker, who initially considered that childhood malnutrition led to higher rates of coronary heart disease in adulthood (Davey Smith, 2003). Forsdahl and Barker both arrived at the conclusion that more powerful than childhood conditions was the nutrition experienced *in utero*. This led to the concept that nutrition and conditions throughout life could affect health, which became known as the life-course approach.

Unfortunately, some approaches can lead to 'victim blaming'. For example, Pitts (1996) highlights the 'Just World Hypothesis', where it is believed that someone brings their own misfortune. She uses the stigma and blame attached to HIV/AIDS, and to diseases arising from smoking and obesity, as an example of this, differentiating between 'innocent victim' and 'thoroughly deserving victim'. The idea of the 'deserving' and 'undeserving' poor is not new, as the Victorians upheld this notion, and the concept of there being a 'morality to poverty' has recently emerged in some media reports (Wynne-Jones, 2013) along with the 'chav' stereotype of the working-class (Jones, 2011). The relevance of this phenomenon to the wellbeing agenda and the work of HWBs is evident in the reflection of the views of local leaders on the balance between individual responsibility and the role of society in tackling health inequalities and the consequent priorities and funding allocations. An example of this was seen at an HWB where there was a historic difference in funding allocations between deprived and more affluent areas in a county, and there was much discussion on how funding could be allocated more fairly, according to local needs.

SOCIAL DETERMINANTS OF HEALTH

Marmot and Wilkinson (2006) describe the 'causes of the causes' of health inequalities as the 'social determinants of health' using the example of smoking contributing to many diseases. The social determinants in this case would not be cigarette smoking, but the reasons why people smoke. Marmot *et al.* (2010: 16) identify the social determinants of health, or causes of health inequalities, as 'material circumstances, the social environment, psychosocial factors, behaviours and biological factors'. This theory recognises that many determinants of health originate 'upstream' and therefore need to be addressed at that level. Such policies by their nature require a multi-faceted approach across agencies and professional groups and are relevant to the role of HWBs; indeed, some commentators expect that services will be planned around the social determinants of health (Peate, 2012). However, in practice they have received less attention than integration of health and social care, which is a primary HWB duty. To illustrate, all HWBs involved in this doctoral research have devoted meeting time to integrated care, whereas very few have been seen to discuss issues such as education, poverty, transport, air quality or housing in any depth, if at all.

As we have seen, the causes of health inequalities are highly complex and they remain the subject of some speculation and ongoing research. As such, they are not straightforward to either define or address and there are difficulties in evaluating the short- and medium-term effectiveness of interventions which may only be apparent in the long term. This can cause problems where funding is based on short-term outcomes and where the electoral system results in pressure to demonstrate policy impacts in one term of office.

Unsurprisingly, there are many suggestions as to what might work in tackling health inequalities. In their review, Marmot *et al.* (2010) suggest six policy objectives. These are:

- Give every child the best start in life
- Enable all children, young people and adults to maximise their capabilities and have control over their lives
- Create fair employment and good work for all
- Ensure a healthy standard of living for all
- Create and develop healthy and sustainable places and communities
- Strengthen the role and impact of ill health prevention.

The Public Health White Paper *Healthy Lives, Healthy People: our strategy for public health* (Department of Health, 2010b) explicitly accepts Marmot's approach. However, this does not include a commitment to the healthy standard of living objective, which relates to minimum income and other financial matters. The majority of HWBs involved in this research had used the life-course approach, as advocated by Marmot, as a framework for prioritisation, with the emphasis generally being placed on children.

There is significant support from others on the need to tackle poverty; for example, Mitchell *et al.* (2000) consider that the number of premature deaths in Britain would decline if there was full employment, a modest redistribution of wealth, and an end to childhood poverty. There is a difference, however, between improving the economic circumstances of the poorest people and creating economic equality in a society. Different countries have adopted different strategies; Japan, for example, has reasonably equal wages, whilst Nordic nations utilise the taxation system to redistribute wealth (Bartley, 2004).

It is evident that there is no agreed approach to tackling health inequalities or the social determinants of health, that they are complex and multifactorial issues and that only a minority can be addressed by the health service (Asthana and Halliday, 2006). We can also see that taking action on some of the social determinants of health is not within the gift of local HWB members and partners. In addition, environmental health, which has a primarily preventative role in improving living and working conditions, has been found to be somewhat uninvolved and overlooked by HWBs, although in some areas practitioners and managers are gaining recognition in HWB sub-structures.

PREVIOUS INITIATIVES AND PARTNERSHIPS

Although the UK has measured, monitored and researched health inequalities for longer than any other country, Johan Mackenbach (2010) points out that the strategies attempted so far have been largely ineffective. This is generally a consensus view, summed up by the White Paper '*Healthy Lives, Healthy People: our strategy for public health in England*', which states that:

> "Health inequalities between rich and poor have been getting progressively worse. We still live in a country where the wealthy can expect to live longer than the poor." (Department of Health, 2010b: 2).

The history of wellbeing as a policy concept is discussed in detail in *Chapter 3*. However, readers may wish to familiarise themselves with former initiatives aimed at health improvement such as Health Action Zones (Mackenbach, 2010), Local Strategic Partnerships (LSPs) (Hills and Stewart, 2005) Healthy Settings (Dooris, 2004) Sure Start Children's Centres and Children's Trusts (Murty *et al.*, 2009), which have often met with limited or patchy success.

Following the major health service and LA restructure of 1974, various efforts have been made to encourage joint working towards common goals (Evans and Killoran, 2000; Smith *et al.*, 2009), with partnership working between these organisations forming a key part of government policy. Joint working was mandated in the Health Act 1999, which requires that NHS bodies and LAs 'cooperate with one another to secure and advance the health and welfare of the people of England and Wales' (HM Government, 1999, Section 27 (1) (1)). However, partnership working between LAs and the health services is not straightforward, as boundaries have not necessarily been coterminous and practices and language can be quite different. Evans and Killoran (2000: 8) found that whilst strategies may need to undertake 'joined up thinking for joined up problems', there is 'a difficult reality of securing integrated action on the ground'. Others add that the historic division between health and social care functions has led to "a series of practical barriers to effective joint working which continue to frustrate service users and staff and to consume significant management time" (Glasby *et al.*, 2010: 245).

Staite and Miller add that there are also significant differences between professional groups involved in HWBs:

> "The differences form icebergs – some are above the surface, but most lie below, unacknowledged, poorly understood and a hazard to effective partnerships. These include differences in roles, language and experience as well as the differences between those who work within the framework of local democracy and those whose political masters are in Whitehall" (Staite and Miller, 2011: 9).

The historical context is also important and the quality of previous relationships can be a factor in determining the ambition of policies (Glendinning, 2002). This observation is very important in relation to HWBs, where this research has found that many individuals are involved who have worked together previously, successfully or otherwise; however, there appears to be a shared enthusiasm in wanting to make the HWB partnerships work.

POTENTIAL HWB IMPACTS ON HEALTH INEQUALITIES

What we can see from the varying explanations for health inequalities is that they have in common the belief that they cannot be tackled solely by medical means.

Action on the social determinants of health was rarely overtly discussed at HWB meetings, which tended to focus on health and social care matters; however, most HWB members were able to talk about health inequalities in interviews and there was a deep commitment from the majority of EH practitioners and managers to tackle the social determinants, which is not surprising given their professional training and background.

HWB members and support officers were generally optimistic about the impact they could have on health inequalities in local populations, as described by a HWB member:

> "I think we'd be expecting to see, with such local control over health, a narrowing of the gap in terms of the health inequalities" (HWB member ID28).

However, these hopes were often linked to very defined areas or issues. A minority felt that the HWB could only have a limited effect, given the impact of social determinants of health outside their remit, as described by an HWB support officer:

> "Addressing health inequalities is bloody difficult. My personal view is I kind of question whether specific actions even make any difference to health inequalities, when you're looking at such a grand scale…. You try and do all this kind of community stuff and get people to go to their screenings, and then unemployment doubles and all the work is washed away within six months." (HWB support officer ID14).

Professor Chris Bentley has expressed concerns that HWBs might be too 'pink and fluffy' and may lack 'firmness or stiffness of spine' to make an impact on health inequalities (O'Dowd, 2013: 1), whilst others felt that 'there is always the danger that HWBs will end up as talking shops' (Sillett, 2012: 710). Some have described a general pessimism about the ability of GPs to commission at a population level and a 'reduced commitment to a health inequalities agenda' (Turner *et al.*, 2013: 1). There were also concerns about how the impact of their work would be attributed and measured, as described by an HWB member:

> "...you can look at what's happening to life expectancy, what's happening to inequalities, what are our immunisation rates doing, but actually which of those bits, if any, are due to the health and wellbeing board?" (HWB member ID11).

Others, such as this elected HWB chair, felt that the wellbeing agenda was already having an impact locally:

> "...I think that word wellbeing has been enormously beneficial, because it means you can test the county transport plan against the wellbeing agenda. What's that got to do with health? Well, if you're going to stop accidents you're going to save the health service a lot of money. Walking routes to school, healthy access to open spaces. It's all part of the same wellbeing agenda. So all local authorities do now is test it against the wellbeing agenda." (HWB member ID10).

EH practitioners and managers often felt that they were not playing as full a role as they could and should be in the new system; however, the majority were hopeful about their ability to adapt and to find a way to link into the public health system as it is established.

CONCLUSION

It should be borne in mind that this research took place during the early stages of HWB development and early functioning and therefore does not enable the evaluation of policies or strategic decisions. It appears that HWB members and EH practitioners and managers have a commitment to tackling health inequalities, although the way that they might go about this task is somewhat unclear in some areas, particularly where the agenda has been dominated by health and social care issues. Whilst we can see that the terminology and concepts around HWBs, wellbeing, and health inequalities are not clear, and inevitably mean different things to different people, there is a willingness and commitment to grasp the opportunities offered by the new structure and working relationships to impact the health of local populations. However, given past initiatives and financial constraints, some are less optimistic about success in tackling health inequalities at a population level.

RESEARCH POINTER 4.1

Look up the Joint Health and Wellbeing Strategy (or equivalent) for your area and note the local issues and priorities.

- Do they include health *and* wellbeing and action on the social determinants of health?

- What could have influenced these local priorities?

- Now compare it to another area with different characteristics; for example choosing an urban and a rural area or an affluent and a deprived area. What are the similarities and differences in priorities? What would you have included in and excluded from these strategies and why?

FURTHER READING

Bartley, M. (2004) *Health Inequality: an introduction to theories, concepts and methods.* Cambridge: Polity Press.

Dorling, D. (2013) *Unequal Health. The scandal of our times.* Bristol: The Policy Press.

Walker, P. and John, M. (Eds) (2012) *From Public Health to Wellbeing. The new driver for policy and action.* Basingstoke: Palgrave Macmillan.

PART TWO

WELLBEING: CONTEXTUALISED

05

THE LIVING ENVIRONMENT AND WELLBEING: WICKED PROBLEMS, WICKED SOLUTIONS?

Jill Stewart and Jim Gritton

AIMS OF CHAPTER:

- To review opportunities to promote housing and wellbeing based on evidence;

- To consider two complex challenges for housing and wellbeing: those living in poor privately rented housing, and those ageing in place;

- To explore some of these complex interrelationships of housing, health and wellbeing in the light of theories around 'wicked' or 'messy' issues.

INTRODUCTION

Housing is an integral part of the wellbeing agenda, and links between housing, health and, more recently, wellbeing are firmly established. Wellbeing emphasises mental and emotional health, as well as enhancing quality of life, where possible, through supportive relationships and active citizenship. Questions about what constitutes wellbeing are considered elsewhere in this book (see *Chapters 2* and *3*). In this chapter we are concerned with some of the pertinent relationships, and complexities around how wellbeing needs can differ according to choices (or lack thereof) and how housing, health and social care needs change across the lifespan.

Evidence indicates that in order to maintain, promote and improve wellbeing, housing needs to be of decent quality, set in neighbourhoods offering community facilities and amenities, with places for children to play and adults to meet in the development of positive social relationships (see, for example, Marmot *et al.*, 2010; WHO and Commission on the Social Determinants of Health, 2008). Our knowledge is moving forward from the relationships between housing and wellbeing, to what we can do about it in practice to support and enhance often complex, multifaceted and sometimes changing housing and social care needs, in ways that are evidence-based and effective (Stewart, 2013).

However, a person's or community's housing is frequently indicative of their socio-economic position in society: is it a person's poverty or their housing environment that causes ill health? Many low income households suffer multiple stressors, which can place additional pressure on their families and communities and over which they may have little, if any, control or even influence (see, for example, Stewart *et al.*, 2005).

We are in a major phase of transition in public health and wellbeing and rethinking how we can best address the social determinants of health. Health and Wellbeing Boards (HWBs) will look to Joint Strategic Needs Assessments (JSNAs) with demonstrable health and wellbeing impacts and outcomes (see *Chapter 4*). As part of the policy context and location in local authorities, those charged with delivering public health and wellbeing will need to develop skills in using datasets to support evidence-based strategies and interventions that are evaluated for effectiveness.

A focus on partnership and evidence-based practice is further consolidating strategies and interventions as Public Health England reiterates the importance of delivering increasingly effective and proactive services, focusing on the social determinants of health to protect, improve and promote health. In housing, health and social care, this requires continued attention to demographic change, stock availability and condition, regard to changing housing need across the life-course, and consolidation of existing service provision to maximise both health impact and health outcomes of interventions and strategies.

As wellbeing becomes embedded as a key part of the public health agenda, with its new organisational and cultural changes, those charged with delivering housing services will need to look to more effective means of engagement in addressing our housing stock, but also in meeting wider wellbeing need. We need to find new ways of intervening in addressing housing stock and the complex lives of those who live there, particularly where alternative housing is frequently neither an option nor a choice in the short or longer term.

This chapter explores two very different manifestations of wellbeing in the housing sector. Firstly it looks at the bottom end of the privately rented sector, where housing conditions and insecure tenure can have a negative effect on wellbeing, and asks how the impact of some of these effects might be mitigated by effective partnership arrangements, particularly where children are involved. It then looks at a very different housing area – that of owner occupiers 'ageing in place' and how housing, health and social care partnerships can work in greater collaboration to provide more effective services in maintaining wellbeing. We then consider so-called 'wicked problems' in housing and wellbeing, using systems thinking and soft systems methodology to get 'under the skin' of some significant wicked issues and the need for effective, evidence-based collaborative solutions.

CAN WELLBEING BE ENHANCED FOR THOSE WITH FEW HOUSING OPTIONS?

As access to housing for many people closely correlates with income, rather than need, those on limited budgets have little choice in their housing. Whilst the privately rented sector caters well for some, at the bottom end it can be expensive, insecure and of poor condition. Many individuals and families can feel trapped in the sector, with little chance of their situation changing, and may or may not be able to access other housing tenures, either social housing (excluded due to ineligibility) or owner occupation (exclusion due to finance or previous inability to fund a mortgage, even though the rental level may be broadly equivalent to mortgage repayment). The focus of this section of the chapter is the lower end of the privately rented sector and it illustrates the challenge of improving wellbeing in the face of so many confounding factors.

The privately rented sector is complex and has disproportionate numbers of mobile and newly formed households, and its tenants tend to have less security than those in the social housing sector (see, for example, Kemp and Keoghan, 2001; Kemp, 2011). It has a high proportion of non-decent homes (Parliamentary Office of Science and Technology, 2011). Since 1988, private sector housing tenancies are 'Assured Shorthold', generally meaning a fixed-term tenancy (often fixed at six months) at a market-based rental level. For tenants, this can be stressful because long-term security is not guaranteed. In addition, there is evidence to suggest that many tenants seeking necessary repair work, etc. may find themselves in a worse position, facing rental increase, harassment or retaliatory eviction (Crew, 2007; Emanuel, 1993).

Houses in multiple occupation (HMOs) which are unsuitable house or hotel conversions can be particularly problematic and of poorest condition. This type of living accommodation includes hostels, houses divided into bedsits, and hotels used as permanent residences. Issues facing residents of this form of shared accommodation are not just related to poor housing conditions and inadequate amenities (bathroom, toilet, kitchen) but they may also be social, and/or emotional, particularly in the case of numerous families with complex needs and chaotic lives (including frequent movers) living in close quarters.

Whilst bedsits can provide low cost accommodation, they may also pose significant risks to the mental health of residents, and contribute to elevated levels of stress, anxiety and depression. Living in bedsits can make it difficult for residents to overcome drug and alcohol problems, often due to the behaviour of other residents (Barratt *et al.*, 2012a). Local authorities vested with improving conditions need to look more widely than just the physical housing conditions to mitigate wider health and wellbeing risks (Barratt *et al.*, 2012b). A further pressure for residents living in what were once hotels, now used for more permanent residence, can be food poverty, as kitchen facilities can be inadequate. Some authorities, such as Thanet District Council in Kent, are seeking to plug the gaps and help support more balanced diets where this applies (Hopkins, 2011).

Physical housing conditions aside, concerns have also been expressed about the Universal Credit and how existing and potential tenants might be able to access and maintain a private sector tenancy, further aggravating some of the health inequalities identified by Marmot *et al.* (2010). The Pro-Housing Alliance Report (2012) found that feelings of insecurity, stress and anxiety, and moving home added to existing problems such as isolation, loss of confidence and debt. Sometimes this meant making stark choices between 'heating or eating'. This report also identified a need to help tenants manage the changes in their lives without further detriment to their health and wellbeing.

Individuals and families with already complex needs may find themselves in this sector, or the sector may aggravate and create additional wellbeing needs. Questions relating to housing and wellbeing seem clear cut: people need somewhere secure, safe and affordable to live. What can services hope to offer those for whom wellbeing seems so out of reach?

Local authorities and their partners charged with enforcing, advising on and advocating for better living conditions in the private housing sector are faced with major challenges. Insecure tenancies and high rents are, to a great extent, out of their remit, but helping to support tenants though streamlined services that include advice and prompt benefit payments can make a real difference, alongside access to more suitable accommodation where this is possible. There are a range of options to help address fuel poverty, providing for warmer homes and potential for additional family income to spend elsewhere. Access into and assistance to remain in housing aside, there are many agencies able to help mitigate some of the negative wellbeing effect of the private housing sector, including Children's Centres which can offer a range of family support. Together with some of the innovative approaches many agencies are offering individually such as subsidised meals, more widely socio-economic regeneration can help provide and support access to education, training and employment opportunities for a more sustainable approach in addressing both individual and community wellbeing.

HOW CAN WELLBEING BE ENHANCED FOR THOSE WHO 'AGE IN PLACE'?

As a population we are living longer, and as we 'age in place', new challenges are presented for policy makers in supporting people to stay in their own homes for as long as possible. Successive governments have encouraged owner occupation as a cornerstone of personal responsibility, and the Government is increasingly looking to owner occupiers to use their own finance, including releasing equity from their property, to maintain, repair and improve their own homes.

As people grow older, the housing conditions may deteriorate around them, particularly if living alone; they are likely to be at home for longer, meaning that it would be more expensive to heat adequately. Added to this, the ageing process may affect their physical and mental health in other ways, with an increasing risk of suffering home accidents and increased likelihood of dementia, each of which has an impact on their housing, health and social care needs.

With the demographics of an ageing population come more degenerative illnesses, and disease, notably dementia, which has become a priority policy area. This is now raising significant questions about the extent to which the State should support people living in their own homes and there are fundamental housing, health and social care implications to be considered. The numbers of people with dementia are increasing and most live in their own homes, more than half of these on their own (see evidence cited in Andrews and Molyneux, 2013).

Helping provide appropriate support to those with dementia in the owner occupied sector, and where applicable their carer (who will also be ageing and have their own developing needs), closely correlates with housing conditions. A healthy living environment remains important, and additional considerations and adaptations will become necessary as the condition deteriorates. With more time being spent at home, the cost of heating and lighting will be greater and there is an increased likelihood of home accidents, as well as a potential increase in isolation and loneliness.

Awareness, early diagnosis, appropriate treatment and signposting to alternative options can greatly enhance quality of life for both the person with dementia and their carer. Home-based solutions can help prevent crises arising and focus more on quality of life, relieving the pressure on number and duration of hospital stays, reducing costs elsewhere in the system (see, for example, evidence and good practice cited in Andrews and Molyneux, 2013). For some years, Home Improvement Agencies have been working to deliver more focused services based on individual need by drawing in appropriate expertise to help minimise disruption and maximise health and wellbeing outcomes for their clients, a role which can continue to be developed into other client areas.

Care and Repair England's 2012 brochure recognises that most people wish, and are able, to stay in their own homes for as long as possible, where the right housing and care support is combined with design and layout changes that take account of dementia symptoms, including memory loss, mood changes and problems in communicating and reasoning. In summary, the brochure suggests that certain features are particularly taken into consideration in supporting someone remaining in their own home (see *Table 5.1*).

With this renewed emphasis on effective partnerships, floating support within dementia-friendly communities will help ensure inclusion, independence and quality of life (Andrews and Molyneux, 2013), and continued research will pave the way for new methods of intervention.

Table 5.1 *Making it easier to keep living at home.*

Feature	Suggestions to make things easier at home
General design and layout	Strong colour coding to enable recognition and recall function; clear spaces to enable safety and mobility as well as ease of finding things; seating near windows for sensory and memory stimulation; glass fronted doors for recognition, with clear containers.
Lighting and heating	Promote strong daylight but reduce glare; good artificial light but avoid shadows; use timers and motion sensitive lights; fit fireguards and easy to use controls with timers and thermostats for water and heating.
Safety and security	Fit smoke and carbon monoxide detectors; install a key safe so trusted people can enter; fit hand and grab rails as necessary; investigate appropriate specialist equipment and adaptations, including telecare such as personal sensors to monitor movement and behaviour and trigger call for help when required.
Retro decorating	Identify items which trigger positive memories across senses of taste, smell, colour, shape and size; use older styles.
Going out and about	External door sensors and reminders; use familiar routes and use tracking devices (or mobile phone with location finder), carry a form of identity.
Gadgets and equipment	Get expert help and advice.

Source: Adapted from Care and Repair England (2013).

HOUSING, HEALTH AND WELLBEING: WICKED ISSUES, WICKED INTERVENTIONS?

In this chapter thus far, we have drawn attention to the complex interplay of housing, health and wellbeing. Many individuals, families and communities have complex, intractable needs that are difficult to address because the causes are deep-rooted and intertwined. Part of the difficulty in tackling such problems is that we often apply solutions that are really only useful for solving simple problems. What can we do about this? Perhaps the first step is to conceptualise the problems differently. Some problems are so persistent, stubborn and difficult to resolve, that they are often described as 'wicked' – not in a pejorative sense but in terms of their resistance to treatment or resolution. Wicked problems have many interlinking causes; they are difficult to categorise or define, and they tend to be immune to 'right' answers or simple solutions. They include many health and wellbeing problems; for example, poverty, mental health, substance misuse, antisocial behaviour or poor housing.

The origin of the concept of a wicked problem is usually attributed to Horst Rittel and Melvin Webber (1973), Professors of the Science of Design and Urban Planning, respectively, at the University of California at Berkeley. Unlike difficult but relatively straightforward problems, which can usually be solved over time using tried or tested methods (these are referred to as tame problems), wicked problems have many interdependent causes, and attempts to find a solution sometimes result in unforeseen or undesirable consequences. Worse still, they may even aggravate the problem. According to Rittel and Webber (ibid.), there are at least ten distinguishing properties of wicked problems and these can be used as a handy checklist for determining whether a problem is in fact wicked:

1. There is no definitive formulation of a wicked problem.
2. The search for solutions never stops with wicked problems.
3. Solutions to wicked problems are neither right nor wrong, but better or worse.
4. There is no immediate or ultimate test of a solution to a wicked problem.
5. Every solution to a wicked problem is a 'one-shot' operation – because there is no opportunity to learn by trial and error, every attempt counts significantly.
6. Wicked problems do not have a calculable or exhaustively describable set of potential solutions.
7. Every wicked problem is essentially unique.
8. Every wicked problem can be considered to be a symptom of another problem.
9. A wicked problem involves many stakeholders, all of whom will have different ideas about what the problem really is and what its causes are.
10. Problem-solvers are liable for the consequences of the actions they generate.

Wicked problems have captured the attention of a number of other theorists, among them Russell Ackoff (1974), erstwhile Professor of Management Science at the University of Pennsylvania, who used the term 'mess' to describe complex problems. Although similar in idea to wicked problems, the main difference is one of nuance: the word mess is used to describe a complex network of interrelated problems that interact with each other. In contrast, Ronald Heifetz at the John F. Kennedy School of Government at Harvard University prefers the term 'adaptive challenge' to describe 'systemic problems with no ready answers' (Heifetz and Laurie, 1997: 124). The challenges are adaptive because solutions require new thinking, experimentation and a preparedness to think outside the box. In this chapter, we treat the three terms as de facto synonyms.

In order to be able to tackle wicked problems, we need to consider them in an all-round context. One way of approaching this is to use systems thinking, which is a holistic approach to analysis that seeks to understand how a system's parts interrelate and influence one another within a larger whole. In order to make sense of a wicked problem, we need to view it as a whole and understand the relationship of the many parts that contribute to the problem's complexity (see *Figure 5.1*).

Tempting as it may be, splitting the problem into parts and analysing each in isolation will not address the whole problem. To misquote Aristotle, a wicked problem is more complex and stubborn than the sum of its parts! In systems thinking, 'a problem is not solved by

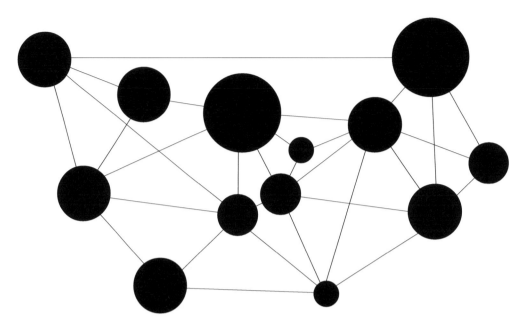

Figure 5.1 *A system has many interrelated parts.*

taking it apart but by viewing it as a part of a larger problem' (Ackoff, 1974: 14). If we use the idiom 'can't see the wood for the trees' as a metaphor, systems thinking is about diverting the focus of our attention away from the trees to the wood that they obscure.

Space precludes a detailed discussion of the origins of systems thinking in this chapter, but it has a long, interesting history which draws from cybernetics, engineering, biology, anthropology, management and many other disciplines too. (For readers who want to know more, *Systems Thinkers* by Ramage and Shipp (2009) is well worth a read.) The important thing to note about the development of systems thinking over the last 100 years is that it is both multidisciplinary and interdisciplinary. This not only highlights the need to view wicked problems from multiple perspectives but also suggests that only collaborative, multi-agency solutions will break down the kind of wicked problems seen in health and social care.

One specific branch of systems thinking that is particularly relevant to the kinds of wicked or messy problems discussed in this chapter is soft systems methodology (SSM), although it was originally developed as a learning system for tackling the wicked problems that managers face in organisational life. As an approach, SSM is most commonly associated with the work of Peter Checkland, Emeritus Professor of Systems, and his colleagues at Lancaster University. Deriving from his work on action research, SSM emerged as an approach for tackling real-world problems, and provides a methodology for dealing with wicked or messy problem situations – "soft systems methodology (SSM) is an organised way of tackling perceived problematical (social) situations. It is action-oriented. It organises thinking about such situations so that action to bring about improvement can be taken" (Checkland and Poulter, 2006: xv).

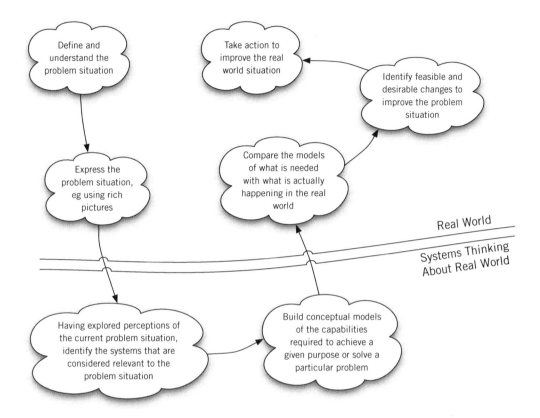

Figure 5.2 *Soft Systems Methodology (adapted from Checkland and Scholes, 1990).*

SSM involves seven stages (see *Figure 5.2*). Although the stages are often represented in linear, sequential fashion, Checkland was keen to stress that they should not be viewed as a constraining straitjacket. Rather, users should feel free to start at any point and complete as many iterations as necessary to gain benefit from the model's use.

One of the most useful techniques drawn from SSM is rich pictures. Sometimes referred to as a situation summary, a rich picture is a flexible, creative and graphical technique, used to depict a complicated or problematic situation. Indeed, a well-crafted rich picture will contain everything that is relevant to a complex situation (see Monk and Howard, 1998, for some useful examples of rich pictures). Although rich pictures may sometimes look like a child's drawings because they contain cartoons or stick figures, the technique is deceptively powerful, as the very act of drawing the picture can reveal important insights about a problem.

One of the things that make wicked problems particularly challenging to deal with is the fact they are socially complex: they involve multiple stakeholders and seldom sit within the jurisdiction of one single organisation or agency. Moreover, stakeholders are seldom a homogeneous group and may have competing needs and/or vested interests. To quote Rittel and Webber (op. cit.: 169), "what satisfies one may be abhorrent to another … [and] what comprises problem solution … is problem-generation for another".

Perhaps not surprisingly, the need for collaboration among stakeholders is a popular refrain in the literature on wicked problems. However, collaboration requires trust, knowledge sharing and structures that facilitate rather than impede the search for collaborative, multi-agency solutions. Sadly, hierarchical structures, bureaucratic cultures, professional 'preciousness' and inward-looking policy making act as a powerful but often invisible deterrent to knowledge sharing and cross-boundary collaboration, a viewpoint shared by Dawes *et al.* (2009: 395): "The boundaries of organisations, jurisdictions, and sectors present the most obvious challenges, but more subtle boundaries related to ideology, professional norms, and institutional divisions can be equally problematic". They go on to argue that success in tackling wicked problems means overcoming a 'need to know' culture in organisations and fostering a 'need to share' culture instead, but how can we achieve this?

David Hunter (2009), Professor of Health Policy and Management at Durham University, calls for a new leadership paradigm, arguing that we need leaders who are more politically astute and who are prepared to confront power and exert influence – "only through such means, and through seeing public health problems as examples of complex adaptive systems, can successful inroads be made into wicked problems" (ibid.: 203). They also need to think and act pro-socially and behave in a way that fosters collaboration and trust. This means building relationships with stakeholders and empowering others within the organisation to do the same, especially those who share clients with partner agencies, because solutions "reside not in the executive suite but in the collective intelligence of employees at all levels, who need to use one another as resources, often across boundaries" (Heifetz and Laurie, 1997: 124). It goes without saying that leaders at all levels of the organisation must be able to distinguish a wicked problem from a tame one. This means developing skills in systems thinking and building a toolkit of methodologies for successfully tackling wicked problems.

CONCLUSION

Many of the most intractable problems in housing, health and social care are certainly wicked or messy in the sense intended by Rittel and Webber (1973) or Ackoff (1974) above. For reasons we have explained, such problems need to be considered in the round using systems thinking, to make sense of their complexity and to facilitate a better understanding of the dynamic relationship between the problem's constituent parts and those whom it affects. This calls for a different way of thinking about and tackling wicked problems predicated on system-wide approaches that involve joined-up working and collaborative, multi-agency solutions (see, for example, *Chapter 8*).

We have seen that housing, health and wellbeing share a complex relationship, and to position housing more centrally, we need to maximise the potential of the new public health and wellbeing apparatus, in particular in demonstrating housing need in JSNAs. Whilst seeing the bigger picture of housing, by learning from and sharing evidence and good practice, and ensuring that the information reaches the right people in influencing policy and strategic direction, we also need to make every intervention count a little bit more.

RESEARCH POINTER 5.1

Read the Joint Strategic Needs Assessment (JSNA) for the area in which you live or work and consider the following questions:

- To what extent is housing considered a social determinant of health?

- How have housing needs been assessed, and why? Are there any gaps?

- What housing issues does the JSNA cover (e.g. overcrowding, availability of open spaces, age of residents, tenure, stock condition, poverty, crime, home accidents, etc.)?

- How will local partnerships deliver wellbeing through housing strategies and interventions?

RESEARCH POINTER 5.2

- What are the housing and wellbeing needs in your neighbourhood?

- How do you know? What evidence do you have to support this?

- Are you aware of where you might access further evidence and examples of good practice to help inform what you are doing, or what your organisation is doing?

RESEARCH POINTER 5.3

- What housing, health or wellbeing problems can you think of that are wicked?

- What makes them wicked?

- What solutions have been tried before, and why haven't they worked?

49

RESEARCH POINTER 5.4

- Earlier we asked you to identify a wicked housing, health or wellbeing problem. Now create your own rich picture that depicts the problem you identified.

- Rather than attempt this on a computer, we recommend you sketch it freehand using symbols, cartoons, keywords, stick figures, arrows and other diagrammatic tools.

- What did you learn about the problem?

FURTHER READING

Hacker, J., Ormandy, D., and Ambrose, P. (2011) Social Determinants of Health – Housing: a UK perspective. In: Porter, E. and Coles, L. (Eds) *Policy and Strategy for Improving Health and Wellbeing (Transforming Public Health Practice Series)*. Exeter: Learning Matters Ltd.

Stewart, J. and Bushell, F. (2011) Housing, the Built Environment and Wellbeing. In: Knight, A. and McNaught, A. (Eds) *Understanding Wellbeing: an Introduction for Students and Practitioners of Health and Social Care*. Banbury: Lantern Publishing.

Stewart, J. and Knight, A. (2011) Private Sector Housing Conditions: Influencing Health and Wellbeing Across the Generations. *Perspectives in Public Health*, 131(6): 255–256. Available online at: **http://rsh.sagepub.com/site/virtual_issues/healthy_homes.xhtml** [accessed 24 March 2014].

06

THE WELLBEING OF GYPSIES AND TRAVELLERS

David M. Smith and Margaret Greenfields

AIMS OF CHAPTER:

- To outline the social, economic and policy factors behind the increasing settlement of Britain's nomadic communities;

- To discuss how the concepts of cultural trauma and collective resilience can aid our understanding of how minority groups respond to external change;

- To examine the relationship between accommodation and the wellbeing of Gypsies and Travellers;

- To explore some of the difficulties faced by newly housed Gypsies and Travellers and consider the impact on subjective wellbeing;

- To consider the role of locally based social networks in boosting individual and collective wellbeing.

INTRODUCTION

This chapter draws on four qualitative studies conducted between 2006 and 2012 consisting of three focus groups and in-depth interviews with 68 Gypsy and Traveller households living in various locations in London and southern England. The aim of the research was to examine their experiences of living in conventional housing. The criminalisation of unauthorised camping, difficulties gaining planning permission for private sites and a decline in public site vacancies following the 1994 Criminal Justice Act have led to an increasing drift into housing over the past 20 years. Around two-thirds of the UK's estimated 300 000 Gypsy/Traveller population is now resident in 'bricks and mortar' (Greenfields and

Smith, 2010).[1] One strand of these studies was concerned with the relationship between accommodation, access to social networks and wellbeing. In this chapter the impact of wider legislative and social factors on the accommodation options and wellbeing of Gypsies and Travellers is considered, and how, through recourse to community networks, external pressures to assimilate are resisted and traditional communal and family structures maintained.

Although they are one of the country's oldest minority groups, the history of Gypsies in Britain is one of prejudice and state-sponsored persecution ranging from policies to exterminate or deport them in the Middle Ages, via policies to eradicate nomadism through removal of children from itinerant families, to forced settlement and assimilation in the modern period (Mayall, 2004). In contemporary society, Gypsies and Travellers remain the most excluded group across several domains: they are the unhealthiest group in society, experiencing more illness and dying younger compared to other minority group members and the lowest socio-economic groups (Parry *et al.*, 2004). Mental health is particularly poor, with a significantly higher percentage experiencing anxiety or depression (32%) than the general population (21%) (Goward *et al.*, 2006). Gypsy and Traveller pupils have the poorest educational outcomes, gaining the fewest GCSEs at grade A*–C; the lowest attendance levels (particularly at secondary school); the highest levels of permanent exclusions and the highest proportion diagnosed with Special Education Needs (SENs) (Cemlyn *et al.*, 2009).

Despite stereotypes associating Gypsies and Travellers with criminality, the Association of Police Chief Officers (ACPO) has stated that they have no more problems with crime among the travelling population than with the general population. However, evidence indicates that they receive unequal treatment by all agencies of the criminal justice system. They are more likely to receive custodial sentences and less likely to be handed community sentences or to be bailed than the general population (Power, 2003).

The marginalised social position of Gypsies and Travellers is a reflection of the extent of societal prejudice that they face. A survey by Stonewall (2003) revealed that more people feel prejudiced towards Gypsies and Travellers (35%) than any other group, followed by refugees and asylum seekers (34%). These perceptions are fuelled by the media, where they are routinely vilified and depicted in ways that would be unacceptable were they directed at any other group (Richardson and O'Neill, 2012). While Gypsies and Travellers do experience high levels of racism, they are more resigned to racial hostility, rarely reporting such incidents to the authorities (Netto, 2008). State officials are not immune from negative stereotyping and reluctance to report racist incidents is grounded in mistrust of the police

---

[1] The figure cited is an estimate of the number of English Gypsies (Romanichals) and Irish Travellers resident in the UK. In addition it is estimated that between 200–300 000 Roma from eastern and central Europe now live in the UK, though many do not declare their ethnicity, making estimating numbers problematic.

in particular, and officialdom in general, and a preference to deal with such problems themselves, which paradoxically entrenches stereotypes of violent criminality. These negative attitudes manifest themselves in a universal desire for spatial separation among the sedentary population. While the 'settled' community demands that nomads cease travelling, there are few issues that galvanise a community as effectively as when opposing Travellers settling in their vicinity, either onto sites or into housing in their neighbourhoods (Ni Shuinear, 1997).

Having outlined the broad social contours within which Gypsies and Travellers live their lives, the following sections will highlight the 'accommodation careers' and experiences of community members in conventional housing, with a focus on wellbeing. This will involve examining the ways in which cultural identities are sustained in the face of a determined assault on their traditional lifestyles and how those identities provide a crucial source of community support that mitigates some of the difficulties faced when dealing with an alien, and frequently hostile, society.

SETTLEMENT, CULTURAL TRAUMA AND WELLBEING

Cemlyn *et al.*, (2009: 5) notes that "in many ways accommodation is key to understanding the inequalities and barriers to services experienced by Gypsies and Travellers". Throughout the 20th and into the 21st century, the impetus behind successive legislation relating to accommodating Gypsies and Travellers has been to settle them either onto approved caravan sites or into conventional housing (Belton, 2005). Government reports throughout the period have frequently stated that the ultimate aim of providing permanent caravan sites was a temporary measure, with the longer-term objective that site dwellers would eventually enter housing. While these aims have been presented in paternalistic terms, Laungani (2002) cautions against the tendency of policy makers to offer universalistic solutions for culturally specific behaviours and preferences. The apparent benevolence of such policies often results in a punitive approach towards groups, who resist being moulded into dominant notions of what is rational and in the group's 'best interests', while the damage that such policies inflict on community members is ignored in a utilitarian pursuit of the 'greater good'.

The growing number of Gypsies and Travellers forcibly settled into housing in the post-war era is relevant to social scientific interest in 'cultural trauma'. This concept has been used by anthropologists and sociologists to account for similarities among a range of indigenous and nomadic communities globally – low educational attainment, high suicide levels, depression, substance abuse and family breakdown – found among peoples who have experienced rapid social change, the destruction of traditional lifestyles and who are widely exposed to discrimination from the economically and socially dominant culture (Tatz, 2004). Cultural trauma refers to events that "leave indelible marks upon their group consciousness" (Alexander, 2004: 1) and contains four elements. First, it has a particular temporal quality and is rapid and sudden; secondly, change is felt deeply and touches the core of the collective order. Thirdly, it is seen as having particular causes that originate from outside the affected group, and finally it is perceived by the group as unexpected, shocking and detrimental (Sztompka, 2004). Evidence indicates that for many Gypsies and Travellers, the move into housing can be traumatic and have a negative impact on psychological wellbeing (Smith and Greenfields, 2013; Parry *et al.*, 2004). This has been recognised in law where the concept of a 'cultural aversion' to housing emerged in a planning case (*Clarke* v. *Secretary of State 2002*) and has been incorporated into guidance regarding assessment of accommodation requirements. Legal judgments following the *Clarke* case state that local authorities should attempt to facilitate a homeless Gypsy's traditional lifestyle by providing a pitch on a caravan site, but if none is available, the local authority can meet its duties by offering conventional housing (Willers, 2010).

For many Gypsies and Travellers the difficulties encountered following initial settlement in housing can be extremely detrimental to psychological wellbeing, which encompasses practical, spatial and social dimensions. For those accustomed to a communal and kin-based existence, not only are many separated from community ties (which also exposes them to an increased risk of racism), but they have to attend to a new set of practical and daily concerns that frequently threaten to "undermine or overwhelm one, or several essential ingredients of culture or the culture as a whole" (Smelser, 2004: 38–40). The following sections will outline some of the practical and social elements of this transition and consider their impact on the research sample of housed Gypsies and Travellers.

HOUSING TRANSITIONS IN 'BRICKS AND MORTAR'

The ethnocentric assumption that equates house-dwelling with improved living standards and enhanced wellbeing is not borne out by research findings revealing the difficulties faced by many formerly nomadic families in housing (Thomas and Campbell, 1992). Budgeting, for example, is a major source of difficulty for those accustomed to daily expenditure patterns. It is frequently the poorer sections of the Gypsy/Traveller community who lack the resources to purchase their own land or private housing (bungalows are the preferred type) that end up in social housing. Two-thirds of respondents estimated that their living standards had worsened since moving into housing, due to higher living costs, which often led families into a spiral of debt (Gidley and Rooke, 2008). One woman recalled that:

> "I couldn't believe the bills ... when I got the bills in I didn't know what to do – we'd only had gas bottles afore that and changed them when they run low. I just ignored the bills until it all got too bad."

Particularly for families with limited literacy, the amount of paperwork and bureaucracy involved in moving into and retaining a property can be overwhelming, sometimes resulting in tenancies being forfeited. While assistance with budgeting and the transition into housing was, in theory, available through 'Supporting People' schemes, these mechanisms were rarely accessed due to previous negative experiences when dealing with officialdom and the anticipation of prejudice and conflict. One respondent argued that:

> "They (officials) don't like Gypsies and they treat you like dirt. We're rejected by some services because they don't want anything to do with us – we need equal rights to be recognised as an ethnic minority and for other people to have more understanding like they do for the others."

Difficulties coping with the practical aspects of life in 'bricks and mortar' are compounded by the unfamiliar physical layout of housing. A sense of spatial disorientation was evident among many respondents, related both to the unfamiliar design of housing, and to the different usage of internal and external living space, which is less distinct for nomadic people than 'settled' communities. Many replicate traditional living arrangements, sleeping communally in one room and making little use of the upstairs. One respondent noted that his family sleep in the living room and "drag the mattresses down at night – upstairs is for the dogs and kids' toys" while another commented that her family were "only using one room and a kitchen – there's too much space in a big house and no real space outside so it's topsy turvy". Indeed the use of outside space for socialising, which was the norm for site residents, could create tensions with their 'settled' neighbours, as such gatherings were often perceived by the latter as threatening and intimidating (discussed below).

Many considered housing as being detrimental to psychological wellbeing, while the contrast between the 'natural' nomadic life and 'synthetic' nature of house-dwelling with its injurious impacts on health was commented on by several participants:

> "Travellers get ill when they go into houses because the air and light are different, it's artificial not fresh air and daylight so a lot of breathing and lung problems start then… Travellers are in housing and living in artificial atmospheres with chemicals and breathing it when they sleep."

A common complaint related to the confined nature of housing and to the physical differences compared to caravans and chalets. These factors exacerbated stress and were accompanied in many cases by claustrophobia and panic attacks, especially among those relatively new to housing:

> "It's just staring at the four walls does my head in. It's terrible, really terrible. I know in a trailer it's smaller but you've got windows all around you and you can see out in all directions who's coming and what's going on so it just feels bigger."

The adverse impacts of housing on the health and wellbeing of Gypsies and Travellers have been well documented. Parry *et al.* (2004) noted that the health of housed Gypsies was poorer than those on sites, with levels of anxiety significantly higher among those in housing. One male observed that:

> "Mental illness is big in the housed Gypsies. I've seen it. It's massive and I see it all through the country. They put them in substandard housing because they think that's what they are, substandard people."

SOCIAL ISOLATION, DISCRIMINATION AND WELLBEING

Practical difficulties of the type described above, and conflict with neighbours had an extremely corrosive impact on the wellbeing of the research sample. The communal and kin-based nature of Gypsy culture has been observed in a variety of historical and geographical contexts, with long-term 'clusters' of different yet related families travelling or living in close proximity to each other the norm (Okely, 1983). Conventional housing – designed for the nuclear family structure – is not always accommodative to this network of extended families, often leaving individual households spatially and socially isolated. When respondents referred to feeling lonely in housing this was generally contrasted to the communal experiences of living on the road and/or on sites, "We miss the site, don't like houses, too lonely, feel too closed in". Social isolation is intensified through hostility from their neighbours and accounts of racism were common, ranging from name calling and repeated and spurious complaints to the authorities, through to physical attacks. One woman described how:

> "the estate's full of unruly kids with no respect, the neighbours are as bad as they used to be. We get hassled all the time with the bad names and we've been broken into many times. Gorjers (non Gypsies) are the worst really badly raised."

Another woman recalled how "they [neighbours] put all the windows out 'cos they found out it was Travellers moving in". Niner (2003) revealed that of the local authorities who responded to her survey, 'problems with neighbours' was one of the main reasons that housed Gypsies and Travellers ended their tenancies, second only to 'inability to settle'. For those who felt "everything is foreign to us - we've grown up in trailers" or who reported feeling "shut in stuck here in this shit house on this shit estate" the absence of social support networks could prove overwhelming, as one woman, discussing the impact of enforced social isolation on her mental health recalled:

> "You'd go literally three months and you might just say good morning to someone outside because they lived their own lives never spoke to each other. I didn't want people in my house but you didn't visit people and it got to the stage when I had the children and post-natal depression kicked in."

As most women were primarily home based they were more likely to refer to social isolation and express concern over loss of family contact after entering housing. One woman observed that "we're all in housing now and it's not our way. It's scattered our people". Parry *et al.*'s (2004) study found higher levels of anxiety and depression among Gypsy women than men, though evidence suggests that the transition from sites into housing has had a negative impact on male working patterns and social status. The study also found that advice workers and community members reported increasing levels of family breakdown and substance abuse following the move into housing (Cemlyn *et al.*, 2009; Smith and Greenfields, 2012). The adverse impacts of housing on individual and collective wellbeing formed the dominant theme in the participants' narratives. However, focusing on the culturally traumatic elements of settlement reveals little about the collective practices and strategies through which settlement and assimilation are resisted and an approximation to traditional communities recreated within housing. These issues are addressed below.

CULTURAL RESILIENCE AND WELLBEING

While the concept of cultural trauma is useful in framing the dysfunctional aspects of social change and its impact on individual and community wellbeing, it only provides a partial view of how individuals and groups respond to fundamental changes in their social environments. The ability to offset external changes through the use of various coping mechanisms will affect how people experience adversity: the fact that Gypsies have survived centuries of persecution and discrimination with their sense of group solidarity and collective identity intact is testament to their resilience. Sutherland (1975) notes that Gypsies represent a prime example of a group that resists enormous pressures to assimilate, managing to live within the wider society, while rejecting its values and institutions. Hollander and Einwohner (2004: 548) highlight the cyclical nature of relations of dominance and resistance whereby "domination leads to resistance, which leads to further domination and so on" which encapsulates the history of relations between nomads and the state. While social, economic and policy-driven factors have combined to restrict the accommodation and lifestyle options of Gypsies and Travellers, these barriers can be overcome through various innovative responses. The following sections will explore how, within a restricted set of options, many community members are able to minimise the impact of changes perceived as antithetical to traditional values.

IDENTITY AND WELLBEING

Social, psychological and developmental studies indicate that a strong ethnic identity generally contributes positively to psychological wellbeing (Madrigal, 2008). Despite the low social status of Gypsies and Travellers, few accept the views attributed to them by outsiders, and their negative profile is continually contested and resisted. McVeigh (1997) notes that in spite of the pervasiveness of anti-Gypsy stereotypes, many Gypsies and Travellers remain convinced of their own superiority vis-à-vis settled society. One way of negating derogatory labelling is through the inversion of stereotypes associating Gypsies with dirt, crime and disorder. These are reversed and levelled at their 'Gorjer' neighbours whose standards of cleanliness and hygiene practices were viewed as inferior to their own. One woman argued that:

> "Gorjers think we're filthy, 'dirty Gypsies' they call us but any Gypsy woman living in a house or a trailer would be ladged (shamed) to keep a dirty place. Our houses are that clean…but the Gorjers round here are that dirty I wouldn't let my dogs use their houses for their toilet."

A further arena where their own practices were regarded as superior to their neighbours was in relation to child-rearing, with different perceptions of anti-social behaviour forming a major source of conflict. One or two related Gypsy families living in the same neighbourhood could result in large numbers of youths gathering outside. This was frequently perceived by the police, social landlords and neighbours as a potential source of disorder. One woman retorted that "that's just our way. It doesn't mean anything and how can we say to [name of son] that he can't see his cousins and friends when they come off the site to call?" Powell (2008: 97) refers to a 'process of collective identification [which] contributes to a 'we image' among Gypsies and a process of disidentification from the settled population". This coheres around attitudes and practices regarding hygiene and child-rearing practices, which place limits on intergroup relations and contribute to the respective groups' ignorance of each other. Intolerance and prejudice foster a willingness to complain to the authorities about Gypsy and Traveller youth, which fuels conflicts between neighbours and adds to the association of Gypsies and Travellers with criminality. As one woman commented, "I hate it here. I haven't got my family here and the police are always at my door". Several participants were critical of their neighbours' parenting skills and their refusal to accept responsibility for their children:

> "They [non-Gypsies] cannot take criticism of their families and if you do complain it'll end up in a fight whereas Travellers they will … sort their kids out when they play up 'cos we all know each other so 'I'll tell our father' normally does it".

Regardless of the length of time spent in housing, 'histories of mobility' and family ancestry are major components of individual and collective identity. Comments such as "we're not born to the houses; we're raised to live in trailers'" were commonplace while the incompatibility of conventional housing with traditional lifestyles and practices formed another aspect of difference and collective identity:

> "Everything is bad [in housing]. Too many bills, don't like the stairs, we can't have a fire in the garden or cook outside or sit outside talking round the fire 'cos the neighbours would call the police. We can't even have family funerals like we would in a trailer."

The possession of a caravan was an important symbol of cultural capital and maintaining the ability to just "get up and go", even if rarely acted upon, could significantly enhance wellbeing. Regulations prohibiting the stationing of caravans outside social housing, or stipulating the length of time that houses can be left vacant placed significant constraints on semi-nomadic practices. Over 65% of those interviewed reported travelling at some point of the year, even if only to attend one or two horse fairs or other culturally important events. A number of parents reported sending their children to spend time with relatives who lived on sites or still travelled to ensure, as one woman said "they don't forget their roots". In other cases a 'rediscovery' of core cultural values and return to traditional lifestyles may feature as a strategy of cultural resistance to assimilation, with an Irish Traveller, for example, noting that "my boys all raised in houses and now they're all on the road. They wanted to live like their grand-folks not like a country person [non-Traveller]". Maintaining a sense of collective identity is essential to individual wellbeing, as a female resident on a private site commented:

> "...the condenseness of the travelling community keeps it alive, without that we'd disintegrate which is what the government want. That'll never happen. Even if they put us all in houses they'll always be who they are."

HOUSING, WELLBEING AND THE RECREATION OF COMMUNITY

Residential concentrations of housed Gypsies and Travellers were identified in all of the study areas, with some estates containing 40–50% Gypsy/Traveller households. In some cases, this was a result of local authority approaches to managing nomadic communities, by moving them en masse into newly built council accommodation following mass evictions or site closures. Another mechanism behind residential enclaves was through an active and conscious approach to the housing allocation system. As priority is given to those with existing family connections in an area, respondents often applied to be housed on estates where a network of relatives were in close proximity. Access to informal sources of knowledge has also enabled a significant degree of movement within housing. A trend of frequent movement between houses was identified as participants exchanged premises through complex networks of carefully planned transfers until they were able to settle closer to their family and wider support system. As one respondent observed:

> "As much as people try to separate Gypsies and Travellers in housing in this area they are wheeling and dealing to be in houses near their own families, so then you end up around this area with estates full of Travellers, and unfortunately people around them don't understand why they want to be together. But it is that family network."

Access to social support networks is a key determinant of psychological wellbeing (Turner, 1981) and in all the study areas, references to the positive aspects of having relatives and/or other Gypsies and Travellers living nearby were prominent: "There are a lot of Travellers round here and that's a good thing because we're in and out of each other's houses". Another participant remarked that "Yeah there are loads of them (Travellers) round here and that's good 'cos we'd go mental otherwise, we have nothing to do with the Gorjers".

Others mentioned the security that comes from being part of a localised and close-knit community, which both expresses and reinforces solidarity:

> "I got family all over this estate. There's so many of us the Gorjers wouldn't dare give us any trouble. That's the best thing about being here, my aunts and cousins are always in our place".

Thus while housing can be experienced as extremely isolating and damaging to wellbeing, the mechanisms through which it is allocated and exchanged mean it can be utilised in a highly versatile manner, facilitating the continuation of community structures and networks in a new context.

CONCLUSION

Bancroft (2005) notes that beneath the heterogeneity of Gypsy Traveller and Roma groups worldwide, the common factors uniting these disparate groups are exclusion and prejudice. While attention has focused either on the small minority with no legal stopping place, who resort to camping in parks and playing fields, or on well-publicised evictions such as from Dale Farm in Essex in October 2011, the plight of those 'settled', often unwillingly, in conventional housing is generally overlooked. Similarly the logic of forcing people into an already severely overstretched supply of social housing, when they are prepared to provide their own accommodation, is rarely questioned. The drive to settlement regardless of human cost raises the question of whether political rhetoric supporting diversity, minority lifestyles and equal rights, is motivated primarily by political expedience and as a diversion from more deep-rooted economic and class-based social divisions.

The settlement of Britain's formerly nomadic communities is also relevant to questions surrounding the role of social support networks in offsetting destructive external pressures and preventing the more damaging impacts of those pressures on individual and communal wellbeing. The concept of cultural resilience is important in comprehending the processes which either assist housed Gypsies and Travellers to adapt, or alternatively to succumb to individual and cultural trauma. For participants, the ability to form spatially bounded networks provided a vital source of support and solidarity which promote wellbeing, while providing a means of both reaffirming collective identity and resisting dispersal and assimilation. These forms of cultural resistance represent 'low profile techniques' through which groups lacking in economic or political power are able to "deny or mitigate claims made by appropriating classes" (Scott, 1985: 302). Indeed, the ability of Gypsies and Travellers to resist policies antithetical to their way of life plays an important symbolic role in raising self-esteem and avoiding the erosion of identity, with significant impacts on the participants' sense of wellbeing.

RESEARCH POINTER 6.1

Go to this generic link which will take you to the most recent caravan count published online: **www.gov.uk/government/collections/traveller-caravan-count.**

- What is the balance between the number of caravans on authorised sites (social rented and private) and unauthorised sites (on land owned by Gypsies and on land not owned by Gypsies) in your region?

- How does this compare with the national picture and how has this pattern changed over the past five caravan counts?

FURTHER READING

Cemlyn, S., Greenfields, M., Burnett, S., Matthews. Z., and Whitwell, C. (2009) *Inequalities Experienced by Gypsy and Traveller Communities: a review.* London: Equality and Human Rights Commission.

Richardson, J. and Ryder, A. (Eds) (2013) *Gypsies and Travellers: Empowerment and Inclusion in British Society.* Bristol: Policy Press.

Smith, D. and Greenfields, M. (2013) *Gypsies and Travellers in Housing: the decline of nomadism.* Bristol: Policy Press.

07

WELLBEING AND OLDER PEOPLE

Anneyce Knight, Vincent La Placa
and Patricia Schofield

AIMS OF CHAPTER:

- To introduce the reader to articulations of wellbeing for older people and their relevance to health and social care practice and policies, particularly with regard to current neo-liberal ideology.

INTRODUCTION

The social construction of ageing is predicated upon the creation of social norms and symbols (both individual and structural) that encapsulates the ageing process and the policy responses to ageing (Powell and Hendricks, 2009). Ageing is perceived as a social and economic challenge, not only for the UK, but also throughout Europe. It is anticipated that by 2025, 20% of Europeans will be 65 and over (European Commission, 2013). In the UK in 2010, the population of 65 and over comprised 20% of the total population and it is estimated that by 2035 this will have increased to 23% (ONS, 2013).

There is no worldwide agreement on the definition of old age. It is generally accepted to be 65 and over in the UK, and is often linked to the age of retirement, but does differ internationally; for example, in Africa, it may be 50 or 55 years old. The World Health Organization (WHO) (2013) suggests that the age of 50 is deemed to be the definition for 'older' and should inform policy making. As definitions of old age remain contested, both policy makers and researchers have employed different definitions.

DEFINITIONS OF WELLBEING FOR OLDER PEOPLE

There is broad agreement throughout this book that there is no consensus as to what constitutes concepts of wellbeing, happiness and quality of life. However, most of the literature posits that wellbeing is constructed on the structural and individual level, and that it can be deconstructed among various interacting domains and processes (McNaught, 2011; La Placa *et al.*, 2013a). For example, the individual, lifestyle, family, community, religion, the dominant economic mode of production, global and national policy discourse.

Debates around wellbeing and ageing have emerged primarily from the fact that the 20th century has witnessed dramatic gains in life expectancy in the UK and much of the developed world. This has been the result of medical innovation as well as enhanced social, economic, and public health innovations that have increased lifespan. This has often meant reframing and developing new policies around 'old age', 'lifespan', 'frail older people' (Tester *et al.*, 2004), 'ageing in place' (see also *Chapter 5*) and 'healthy life expectancy' (Allen, 2008), as new political and cultural concepts have emerged.

Physiological definitions have merged with developing social and political ones, precipitating new responses to old age. The concept of 'life-stage' has also emerged as a discrete entity through which to analyse how individuals construct health and wellbeing in interaction with their social and economic environment according to age, environment and its effects (La Placa *et al.*, 2013b). Other policies, including enhanced interest in gaining consumer views of health care, the emergence of evidence-based medicine requiring outcome indicators, and pressure to augment resource use efficiency, have also contributed to this process.

Another contribution to new discourses around wellbeing and old age is the emergence of neo-liberalism within dominant policy discourses (Stedman Jones, 2012). Neo-liberalism is best captured generically as an ideology that emphasises free markets, reduced welfare expenditure, and individual responsibility for welfare, as opposed to collective provision and wealth redistribution; and the primacy of the individual in making economic choices as opposed to state intervention. This has displaced former post-war consensus discourses around, for example, wealth redistribution, and the belief that older people comprise a category requiring collective provision in the form of state pensions and state provided care. Rather it has been assumed that the free market provides adequate solutions and future generations should be more responsible for financial and personal wellbeing in old age. Neo-liberalism came to the fore in the UK with the election of Margaret Thatcher in 1979. Her government was committed to a radical structural and economic overhaul of society, with much of it centred on reduction in collective social provision.

However, as La Placa and Knight have argued in *Chapter 3*, Thatcherism (and its incorporation of neo-liberalism) was as much a moral and discursive phenomenon, as it was material and economic. Thatcherism had a major impact on changing definitions and articulations of wellbeing for older people. For instance, care of older people was affected by discursive changes, and changes to services, that shifted from 'institutional' to 'community' care in the 1990s (Johns, 2011). Efforts were made to keep older and vulnerable people at home in the community and out of institutional care. This entailed giving older people more choice over care, enabling the private sector to care for individuals within the home, and reducing state care/interventions in older people's lives. The main impact upon wellbeing for older people has been the concept of 'normalisation', that older people should be as much a part of the community as anyone else. However, John (2012) argues that a society organised around the individual and the free market can fail to recognise the contribution that older people have and can have on society. Rather, older people have often been depicted as a financial burden on those in work, impacting negatively on the wellbeing of both.

On the other hand, rising house prices, private pensions and lower rates of inflation since 1979 have enriched many of today's retirees and pensioners, enhancing wellbeing in retirement (Willetts, 2010). However, it must also be acknowledged that other factors, for example demographic and lifestyle changes, are as important as political ideology. This requires a longer-term rethink of policy towards older people and its impact upon discourses of wellbeing in a free market economy.

OLDER PEOPLE, WELLBEING AND QUALITY OF LIFE: CHALLENGES AND OPPORTUNITIES

2012 was the European year for 'Active Ageing' and solidarity between generations. Active ageing in this context is perceived as growing old in good health as a full member of society, feeling fulfilled in employment, independent in everyday life, and involved as citizens (Europa, 2013). These definitions and concepts associate directly with McNaught's definitional framework of wellbeing (McNaught, 2011; La Placa *et al.*, 2013a) in that one can see a multidimensional view, transcending subjectivity, and interlinking with wider determinants. It should also be noted that older individuals are not homogenous in terms of, for example, age, physical health, health and wellbeing, and ethnicity (Knight and Stewart, 2013). There are many generic challenges to healthy ageing, including:

- increasing morbidity and co-morbidity; for example, long-term conditions such as cancer and mental health issues including dementia and depression
- age discrimination
- poverty, including fuel and food poverty
- social exclusion; for example, access to transport and social isolation
- housing; for example, suitability, availability and housing options
- ethnicity and culture.

CASE STUDY 7.1

Ageing well in Europe: the situation in France

Much of the above is similarly identified in Europe. For example, in France, 'ageing well' and 'welfare' in ageing have been watchwords for successive French governments for over 20 years. Life expectancy is higher in France than the European average and is still increasing slightly. Life expectancy without disability remains stable, which suggests that these 'extra' years of life can be lived without limitations to an individual's quality of life.

However, the challenges of 'ageing well' have changed. For example, the development of Cancer and Alzheimer plans means that two major dimensions are now being taken into consideration; the quality of life in the ageing population and ageing in place are recognised and it is acknowledged that society needs to adapt to an ageing population. More recently still, when speaking in France of 'successful ageing', one is talking about a having a 'good death' or 'dying with dignity'. So, in addition to the social questions of ageing well with a decent income (pensions or social allowances), and in decent living conditions, there is the 'ageing well ethic' which involves professionals, families and carers, and the older people themselves.

Quality of life and wellbeing often go together, but the correlation between wellbeing and income (often derived from a pension, or contributions related to working life and employment), as well as the state of health and involvement of the citizen open up new discussions. The 'age-friendly environment' now constitutes a new area of involvement for local and regional authorities. Regarding special needs housing, social contacts, mobility, secure neighbourhoods, work is under way but now requires strong mobilisation of resources, in particular the finance to sustain these. At a time of budget constraints and changes in political philosophies, are the needs of the retired always taken into account?

In the face of structural changes to pension systems and to healthcare, senior citizens are worried. Pensions will fall in value, the indexing will no longer be sufficient, conditions of access to pensions will require more qualifying years of work. One can therefore fear some 'poverty' in old age and at the same time a loss of public confidence in the French system of social security.

Given the demographic evolution of 'live longer, but more alone', even if we see four or five generations coexisting, the temptation is to 'build the right' for each category of citizen, rather than making available 'fundamental rights' to them at all stages of life. The challenge of social cohesion will be answered in protecting older and vulnerable people, in developing neighbourhood solidarity and closeness and in constructing and encouraging a more intergenerational co-existence.

With thanks to Jean-Pierre Bultez, Vice President, AGE Platform Europe/Les petits frères des Pauvres (France).

Older people themselves identify significant factors that influence their ability to cope with ageing. These include the ability to adapt to ongoing physical changes, participating in relationships, maintaining independence, taking risks, having enough money, achieving their desires and personal goals, leading a full life, and participating in meaningful activities (Social Care Workforce Research Unit, 2005).

With such diverse expectations and needs, and difficulties in establishing a precise definition of wellbeing, a more specific focus on older people is required. Much of the emphasis to date has been on mental health and wellbeing. For example, the European Pact for Mental Health and Wellbeing (European Commission, 2008) mentions the need to improve housing and care home design to ensure features are included to improve quality of life and wellbeing for older people; for instance, for those with dementia (Stewart and Knight, 2011). The role of professionals such as environmental health practitioners in providing positive working and living environments to promote wellbeing and mental health is also seen as key (Spear et al., 2011).

The challenge of developing definitions of wellbeing, happiness and quality of life for older people lies in the ability to produce holistic concepts of wellbeing, age and care, which take account of the heterogeneity of older people, the physiological process of ageing, and the structural conditions that afford opportunities and constraints in developing policies and delivering services that enhance wellbeing. This requires an outlook that focuses on subjective/individual and structural issues for older people, and awareness that experience of old age is often mediated by other processes such as lifestyle, preceding life-stages, culture, current demographics and policy paradigms. As Larkin (2013) points out, some of these can be conceptualised as 'protective effects'; for example, an individual who looked after his or her health in preceding years might extend this process to later years; whilst others can constitute 'risk factors', for instance, alcohol consumption, weight gain and lack of sleep (often associated with the physiological process of ageing).

As a result, we advocate that wellbeing policies and interventions around 'older' and 'frail' individuals be developed around 'care', 'compassion' and 'quality of life' for older people, concepts intrinsic to service planning and development for older people (Kydd, 2009). We believe these concepts can apply on individual and structural levels. For example, degrees of care, compassion and quality of life are influenced by structural conditions such as social attitudes to older people, the economy and policy responses to old age. Nevertheless, older people are often autonomous individuals who identify wishes as regards their care, and make choices, which can constitute either protective or risk factors (although it must be acknowledged that in cases of, for example, dementia or severe physical disabilities, choices and capability to act can be severely limited, requiring different responses).

As Kydd et al. (2009) argue, care is constructed around the requirements of older people and embedding these requirements into the planning and delivery of care services and systems – the structural conditions. Care should also be continually delivered with regard to personal needs and the perception of the contribution the individual makes to the family, community and wider society. This is something that the personalisation agenda seeks to address (Community Care, 2008; SCIE, 2010). Quality of life may be applicable to personal and individual definitions of care and wellbeing as defined by older people and those who care and provide services/interventions for them. For example, McKevitt and

Wolfe (2002) compared professional with patient perspectives of quality of life of older patients who had suffered a stroke. They found the professionals adhered to two definitions; one a colloquial everyday sense of 'happiness'; and second a scientific model that could be used for research to rationalise delivery of health care. Older patients who had suffered a stroke defined quality of life in broader and subjective terms, such as ability to participate socially with friends and family; to cook and clean; as happiness, and access to sufficient material resources (McKevitt *et al.*, 2003). However, whilst we have allocated each example to the structural and individual level in this case, a holistic interpretation of wellbeing would view how both levels, and the individuals involved, are interactive and feed off one other. For instance, delivery of services and structures of care can be influenced by patient and professional constructions of care, wellbeing and quality of life. If professionals perceive care and quality of life as largely related to physical health, this can affect delivery of services and routine care which may conflict with patients' views. How professionals measure or assess quality of life and care can have implications for how concepts of wellbeing, care and compassion are reflected in services, both formally and informally.

WELLBEING, POLICY AND SERVICE DELIVERY

National policies have been produced to enhance and equalise care; for example, the National Service Framework for Older People (Department of Health, 2001) and the National Institute of Health and Clinical Excellence (NICE, 2006) guidance for quality in dementia care. Despite this, it has been identified that high quality services are not always delivered to older people, thus impacting on individual wellbeing; for example, the final report of the public inquiry into Mid Staffordshire Foundation Trust (Francis, 2013) identified that older patients had experienced poor care. The Care Quality Commission's (CQC) reports on dignity and nutrition also draw attention to the lack of safe and good quality care for older people (2011; 2013a; 2013b). The Sir Roger Bannister Health Summit in March 2012 highlighted not only the needs of frail older people, and that services should be delivered to meet those needs, but also that often those caring for older people operate within material and employment contexts that comprise low wages and poor working conditions, both in care homes and hospitals, which can affect delivery of services. Many staff have limited qualifications as currently there is no 'gold standard' qualification for health and social care assistants and no regulatory bodies for them, such as those for nurses (Nursing and Midwifery Council) and social workers (Health and Care Professions Council). Both the NHS and higher education institutes, such as the collaboration between University Hospital Southampton NHS Foundation Trust and Southampton Solent University, are seeking to up-skill the non-regulated healthcare work force. This provision is offered at academic level four and five via a unique curriculum which enables clinical learning in a specific specialism, development of compassionate care, and work-based learning which is credit-rated as either Continuing Professional Development (CPD) units of study or as a complete Foundation Degree in Health and Social Care. This 'hub and spoke' model is now being rolled out across the Local Education and Training Board (LETB) area of Health Education Wessex and includes six NHS Trusts, both within hospital and community settings, including mental health and children's care, and is seen as an exemplar of good practice.

Furthermore, the Willis Commission report (2012) into the education of nurses identified that as people are living longer, they require more complex care, and that this should be delivered in a "respectful way, maintaining dignity and wellbeing, and communicating effectively... [to] protect their [patients'] safety and promote their wellbeing" (Willis Commission, 2012: 13). This emphasises a strong correlation between caring and wellbeing. The publication of the '6 Cs' – Care, Compassion, Competence, Communication, Courage and Commitment (Department of Health and NHS Commissioning Board, 2012) – and the subsequent implementation plan have a focus on helping people to stay 'independent', maximising wellbeing and improving health outcomes (NHS England, 2013). Much of the focus recently has been on hospital care. However, Jeremy Hunt MP, as Secretary of State for Health, has recognised that there is a need to improve primary and community care. The proposed new Care Bill seeks to put wellbeing and compassion at the heart of health and social care provision (Hunt, 2013; HM Government, 2013).

Gilbert (2013) also identifies that caring is associated with wellbeing and that being 'helpful' and 'supportive' are at the core of compassion. He suggests that caring involves attending to others' needs and includes ways of thinking about how to be helpful and non-judgmental. In addition, it requires feelings, concern for others, empathy, kindness and warmth, and behaviour that alleviates suffering or helps people to prosper, flourish and grow. Gilbert (2013) argues that compassion has two dimensions, self-compassion and compassion for others. The components of an act of compassion involve noticing, thought and action.

As a result, we believe there is a requirement to develop, for instance, courses in compassionate care for those working with older people in health and social care, as compassion is a value and a skill, learnt through interactions and relationships. The use of the humanities and social sciences such as philosophy and psychology, anthropology, sociology, art and literature, in the form of narratives to underpin a wider perspective beyond the biomedical model, affords opportunities not only to explore the concept of compassion, but also to provide personal development and insight about the resources needed for compassionate care (such as dignity and respect) and an understanding of the service users' needs. For example, individual NHS Trusts and Universities, such as Dartford and Gravesham NHS Trust and the University of Greenwich, have sought to deliver a multi-professional Health Humanities course to address this issue.

The New Economics Foundation's (NEF) (2008) 'Five Ways to Wellbeing' model might also be a suitable framework to incorporate concepts of care, compassion and quality of life adequately. The five ways to wellbeing are: 'Connect', 'Be Active', 'Take Notice', 'Keep Learning' and 'Give'. The framework enables healthcare professionals to design and embed evidence-based wellbeing strategies, according to the needs of a particular group. The Five Ways to

Wellbeing were formulated by the NEF from evidence gathered in the UK government's Foresight Project on Mental Capital and Wellbeing and draw upon extensive research about mental capital and mental wellbeing through life. The Five Ways can be employed to develop organisational strategies, to measure impact, to assess need, for staff development, and to help people to incorporate more wellbeing-promoting activities into their lives.

The concept of 'connect' locates development of relationships with significant others, such as families, friends and across local communities. In terms of older people, this can assume the form of the grandparenting role, where grandparents play a key role in the rearing and socialisation of their grandchildren. Older individuals often refer to grandparenting as a source of pleasure and purpose (Lee, 2006). The idea that wellbeing is enhanced by being 'active' is fundamental to the model and encourages older people to participate in physical exercise and recreational activities. These can range from participation in walking clubs to doing Tai Chi, where there is a growing body of evidence supporting its use; for example its positive cardiovascular effects (NHS, 2012). The importance of local communities' recreational and environmental facilities is emphasised in the Healthy Foundations Life-Stage Segmentation model, as they tend to embed health and wellbeing within locally accessible resources, which are responsive to local people's needs (Williams et al., 2011; Smith et al., 2011; La Placa et al., 2013b). The Silver Line, launched in 2013, seeks to connect individuals to both support services and activities within their local communities (The Silver Line, 2013).

Capacity to take notice can encourage individuals in awareness of their surroundings, whilst developing reflective capacities (such as mindfulness or a sense of spirituality) around enhancing personal and community wellbeing (Knight and Khan, 2011). Older people can be encouraged to develop friendship networks and other relationships that facilitate and enable wellbeing. 'Keep learning' accentuates the need to keep mentally active by, for instance, finding new hobbies and interests. The emphasis is on maximising wellbeing through enjoyable activities that equip older people with new forms of social capital, as well as enjoyable skills-based and leisure activities. Increasingly, older adults are taking on further academic study, compensating for a lack of educational attainment in their youth, or learning a new skill that they had no time for when working. The U3A (University of the Third Age) is a successful movement where retired and semi-retired people can learn from each other and share their knowledge and expertise, either to gain qualifications or for the pleasure of learning (U3A, 2013).

The aspect of 'giving' is articulated within the context of individuals and communities, and the rewards attained through engaging in social activities, for instance, volunteering. Volunteering is associated with enhanced life satisfaction and often enhances mental health in older people (Allen, 2008). It enables them to participate in the life of the community and improves morale and self-esteem (Surr et al., 2005). It can often ease the transition between working life and retirement.

The Five Ways to Wellbeing model is relevant to our view of wellbeing in that it enables older people and service users to articulate definitions of wellbeing, incorporating concepts of happiness, quality of life and care. The model can also strategically operate on the individual and structural levels, enabling development of a host of upstream wellbeing interventions on the macro and individual level. For example, healthcare professionals in charge of care and services can examine the processes that affect experience of services, and find new ways to enhance its responsiveness.

NEO-LIBERALISM, OLDER PEOPLE AND WELLBEING

Previously, we argued that broader ideological developments have impacted upon definitions of wellbeing for older people and responses. For example, the advent of neo-liberalism and, since 1979, Thatcherism, placed emphasis on free markets, competition and individualism, as enhancing personal and economic wellbeing throughout life-stages. It also changed the concept of older people from a category requiring collective assistance, to one where self-reliance and individual provision became applicable. From this perspective, older people were perceived as little different from people of other ages. In fact, the pervasiveness of neo-liberalism normalised older people as an intrinsic part of the community with similar interest in maximising wellbeing through choice, markets and individual preferences.

Neo-liberalism has tended to ideologically and discursively integrate the social category of 'older people' within other mainstream sub-groupings, neglecting the fact that physiological old age, and cumulative risks, may require a more specific focus on their needs and service requirements. Concepts of life-stage, health and wellbeing, and quality of life for older people, are different from other groups, and cannot always be normalised or homogenised with that of the mainstream population. In fact, we believe it is ironic that in emphasising choice, competition and the market, neo-liberalism can end up producing normalised and essentialist categories of individuals, lumped together.

Neo-liberalism may be a dominant framework in developing and applying policy in the UK generally, but this should not imply that it is the only relevant theoretical or epistemological standpoint for approaching wellbeing and old age. As Larkin (2013) points out, old age is often characterised by physical and cognitive changes which are accompanied by deterioration in health and wellbeing. These physical and emotional changes, as well as the design and delivery of services to respond to them, often require different solutions on various levels. Perhaps this too can be perceived as wicked problems requiring wicked solutions (see *Chapter 5*). The wellbeing of older people requires that we focus upon the contexts and events specific to this component of the life-course (whichever way later life is defined or begins). It requires focus upon the wellbeing of older people at the individual and structural levels, including service delivery planning and how this interacts with healthcare professionals' and their definitions of, for instance, quality of life and quality of care (even if this occurs within a generic ideological and economic neo-liberal framework).

This is not to suggest that neo-liberal theory is completely irrelevant to the wellbeing of older people, despite the fact it has tended to homogenise needs and requirements. The decline of class as a useful construct in social analyses has witnessed the emergence of a focus upon consumption processes (Llewellyn, 2009), the processes through which consumer markets integrate individuals into the economy and society. The emphasis is upon how commercialism, consumerism and choice can be advanced for the benefit of older people, when accounting for, for example, delivering travel, recreation and social services, care and housing. Neo-liberalism may be limited in its capacity to define the needs and requirements of older people, but it can point the way to the provision of person-centred and diverse services that respond to needs. The introduction of localism, choice and competition into the construction and delivery of healthcare services can also be seen as part of this consumption process.

As La Placa and Knight (2014) argue, the decentralisation of health and wellbeing policy to local levels and local communities can enable those very communities to design, construct and embed concepts of wellbeing and quality of life at the local level. This would equally apply to the construction and embedding of local policy and discourse around older people's wellbeing. Whilst access to consumer markets, products and services may constitute a more reliable indicator of socio-economic status than traditional concepts of class, one needs also to recognise that reconciliation with neo-liberal theory means not forgetting the fact that consumption patterns vary between different groups, reflecting differential power and economic status. Furthermore, as La Placa and Knight have also argued in *Chapter 3*, this means that constructing concepts of wellbeing often entails accounting for competition for scarce resources and status among social, economic and ethnic groupings. It also means focusing upon how social groups construct different concepts of wellbeing, in relation to and in competition with one another. Context, environment and competition are significant as opposed to 'one size fits all' national definitions of wellbeing.

CONCLUSION

This chapter has focused upon definitions of ageing and wellbeing of older people. Enhanced lifespans, new public health innovations and the emergence of neo-liberalism have changed the ways that we look at older people and their needs, and provide for them. Wellbeing requires an outlook that focuses on individual / subjective and structural levels and awareness that experience of old age is often mediated by other processes such as lifestyle, preceding life-stages, culture, current demographics and policy paradigms. Wellbeing policies and interventions around 'older' and 'frail' individuals should be developed around concepts of, for example, 'care', 'compassion' and 'quality of life' for older people, concepts we believe are intrinsic to service planning and development. It has also alerted the reader's attention to the fact that neo-liberalism can be somewhat limited in its ability to articulate the diverse needs and requirements of older people, due to its normalising and homogenising tendencies.

However, on another level, its emphasis upon choice and diversity of services may make it useful to the design and delivery of services.

RESEARCH POINTER 7.1

- What might be the most important elements in wellbeing for older people?

- Now think of what might be significant elements of wellbeing for older people who have experienced a stroke and/or dementia. Would it be different from the above?

- How could individual wellbeing for people with dementia or those who have suffered a stroke be enhanced?

FURTHER READING

Allen, J. (2008) *Older People and Wellbeing*. Available at: **www.ippr.org/publication/55/1651/ older-people-and-wellbeing.**

Joseph Rowntree Foundation (JRF) (2013) *A Better Life; Old Age, New Thoughts*. Available at: **http://betterlife.jrf.org.uk/?gclid=CJDz7cq2kbsCFa-WtAodQksAiA.**

Macková, M. (Ed.) (2013) *Long Term Care of the Elderly*. Pardubice, Czech Republic: University of Pardubice.

08

BLUE SPACE AND WELLBEING

Anneyce Knight, Jill Stewart, Maureen Rhoden,
Nevin Mehmet and Lynn Baxter

AIMS OF CHAPTER:

- To provide a background to why some once 'health-giving' seaside towns are now struggling to provide an environment conducive to wellbeing;

- To explore selected aspects of a study into how living in private rented accommodation in the seaside town of Margate contributes to family and community wellbeing;

- To discuss McNaught's (2011) holistic framework for wellbeing and its usefulness for research of this nature;

- To consider what seaside towns offer families and communities, including a focus on the built environment;

- To examine a multi-disciplinary approach to enhancing family and community wellbeing.

INTRODUCTION

Britain's seaside towns are varied in character and developed rapidly as Georgian and Victorian holidaymakers began to benefit from easier travel, particularly with the emergence of the railways. As some of the working classes achieved paid holiday leave by the early 20th century, seaside towns further developed to cater for this need by providing entertainment venues.

However, more recent years have seen an increase in package holidays abroad and a subsequent decline in the British seaside town, and many have struggled to regenerate socially and economically, providing major challenges for local and national policy makers and changes to the built environment. As hotels and guest houses have lost much of their traditional income, many have attracted low income individuals and households living in the accommodation on a more permanent basis. This now presents major challenges for the local environment and service delivery as well as for individual, family and community wellbeing.

THE BACKDROP: MARGATE

Margate is located on the north coast of Thanet, Kent, UK with a population of approximately 40 000 (Margate Renewal Partnership, 2009). Historically, Kent has had an important place in the seafaring history of the UK; for example, Chatham dockyards were an important home for the Royal Navy from the 17th century until well into the 20th century, when the number of naval bases was reduced. Margate was originally a small fishing village that developed initially as a small port and became England's first resort to offer a sea-bathing hospital with its reputed health-giving environment. It then developed into a popular British holiday seaside town in the 19th and 20th centuries with a successful tourist economy (Kent County Council, 2011a). British seaside towns have long been associated with promoting health and recreation, thereby enhancing wellbeing. The popularity of Margate has declined since the advent of easier worldwide travel, package holidays, and the loss of the attraction Dreamland, the theme park which had been seen as the 'physical and emotional heart' of the town for over 100 years, resulting in the downturn in the local economy (Margate Renewal Partnership, 2009).

The extent of the level of decay of the built environment is often hidden, with vulnerable areas being part of larger administrative units, which makes their vulnerability less visible. The 2010 Indices of Multiple Deprivation shows that within Kent there were three Lower Super Output Areas (LSOAs) in the top 100 in the country (LSOAs are areas with 1000–3000 people living in them; average population of 1500 people). The areas in this study, Margate Central and Cliftonville, have been ranked nationally 22nd and 33rd, and within Kent first and second (Kent County Council, 2011b). Indeed, Walton and Browne (2010) have confirmed that deprivation has been hard to shift within coastal towns such as Margate and have identified that "…regeneration, in this sense of reviving and revitalising rather than destroying and replacing should generally be the order of the day at the British seaside" (ibid.: 65).

Evidence in a review of coastal towns identified that seaside towns have faced a variety of economic challenges leading to deprivation and subsequent impact on wellbeing. These include:

- Physical isolation, which provides a barrier to economic growth and regeneration
- Low wages, low skill economy and seasonal employment
- High dependency on a single industry
- Outward migration of young people seeking better employment prospects

- Transient populations with so called 'social dumping', often of vulnerable adults and children and asylum seekers
- Higher than average older population with potential additional health and social care needs
- Poor transport infrastructure
- High incidence of poor housing conditions combined with a shortage of affordable housing to buy, higher number of care homes and houses of multiple occupancy (HMOs), and a larger amount of private rented accommodation.

(Source: House of Commons Communities and Local Government Committee, 2007: 8–21)

For Margate, many of the issues identified above are evident. There are high levels of child poverty, a high number of older people, inward migration of vulnerable groups, particularly from European Union (EU) accession countries, high levels of unemployment, HMOs and "a larger proportion of people living with multiple deprivation" (Margate Renewal Partnership, 2009: 1). Consequently, Margate, as with other seaside regions, faces the challenges of addressing the key issues resulting from poverty, health inequalities and social exclusion, with their negative effects on not only health but also the wellbeing of the population (Knight, 2009). Some seaside towns, such as Margate, which have depended on a seaside industry for so long, have particularly suffered. The large and elegant façades of the commercial hotels and guest houses no longer provide a tourist function; they are the smokescreen for Houses of Multiple Occupancy (HMOs) for those on low income and benefit-dependent households within a concentrated area, often with poor quality accommodation. Ironically, the once derelict Royal Sea Bathing Hospital has been converted into luxury apartments by local entrepreneur, Jane de Bliek, and is an example of an initiative to improve the local built environment as recommended by English Heritage and Urban Practitioners (2007).

WELLBEING IN RESEARCH

Wellbeing is now a commonly employed concept, whether by academics, public sector employees, the 'wellness' industry or the press and it is no surprise that to some people it appears to be a very nebulous concept. Wellbeing has often been seen to be tied in with health or as an add-on. As discussed in earlier chapters, current attempts at defining wellbeing are exploring the concept as a separate and more complex notion as, in reality, health is only one component of wellbeing, and the term itself seeks to take the focus away from the biomedical model (Knight and McNaught, 2011). McNaught (2011) suggests that wellbeing is far more than 'feeling good' or 'happy' but has both subjective and objective elements. He provides a structured framework for defining wellbeing which has four different dimensions – individual, family, community and societal (McNaught, 2011). La Placa et al. (2013a) suggest that this multi-level and inclusive definitional framework enables the uniqueness of wellbeing to be explored, both subjectively and objectively, as it "brings together how people feel about their circumstances and assessment of how their objective circumstances affect them as individuals, families and societies" (La Placa *et al.*, 2013a: 120).

McNaught (2011) affirms that individual and family wellbeing are closely linked because the majority of individuals "live within the context of a family (however defined) and the quality of personal relationships and the access to physical and other resources are generally a feature of personal and family wellbeing" (McNaught, 2011: 13). McNaught (2011) further states that there is a range of resources that enhance family wellbeing including child care, sharing resources for daily living, and providing or facilitating economic opportunities for family members; and that both internal and external factors have an impact on the wellbeing of family members (McNaught, 2011: 13). Families normally sit within communities which may be based on factors such as geography, ethnicity or culture. Furthermore, McNaught (2011: 14) proposes that community wellbeing can be seen as a concept which recognises "the social, cultural and psychological needs of people, their family, institutions and communities", which means that other factors, beyond that of subjective wellbeing, need to be considered such as health, poverty, environment, housing and economy.

This framework provides a useful tool to underpin the study that was undertaken in Margate and aimed to explore tenants' reasons for living there from the perspective of those delivering front-line services. The study took place in 2011 and had a specific focus on how living in private sector rented housing impacted upon family and community wellbeing. The research included a desktop analysis of the area and related documents and eleven semi-structured interviews were conducted with front-line practitioners from a variety of backgrounds including environmental health, housing, children's services and the voluntary sector. Their perspectives and experiences were recorded and field notes taken. Ethical approval was sought and agreed. Selected aspects of this study are discussed here.

WELLBEING IN PRACTICE
Living in a seaside town – what do seaside towns offer families and communities?

British resorts, such as Margate, are unable to compete internationally in terms of climate, but do have the advantages of having an attractive landscape along with a solid heritage, which is founded on local architecture, culture and entertainment (Walton and Browne, 2010). Indeed, the seaside has long been associated with a sense of individual wellbeing; for example, the positive perception of a visit to the seaside is enshrined in the popular music hall song of 1907 "Oh! I do like to be beside the seaside. I do like to be beside the sea! I do like to stroll upon the Prom, Prom, Prom! Where the brass bands play: Tiddely-om-pom-pom! So just let me be beside the seaside. I'll be beside myself with glee". More contemporarily, Depledge and Bird (2009) discuss the development of the 'Blue Gym' programme, which aims to persuade people not only to undertake physical activities to promote their health and wellbeing, but also to appreciate Blue Space. Indeed, recent research by the European Centre for Environment and Human Health has concluded that of all the outdoor opportunities, visits to the seaside had the most positive impact on wellbeing (Ashbullby and White, 2012). The reasons for this may be linked to social and/or cultural factors or more intrinsic motivations connected to pleasant childhood memories; hence, the desire for many to live 'beside the sea'. Indeed, the House of Commons Communities and Local Government Committee report (2007: 60) identified that Margate "had a lot to offer tourists and private investors as… Margate was an attractive seaside town with the best beaches".

In the wards of Cliftonville and Margate Central, a variety of reasons for living in the area were cited in the interviews. Many of these front-line practitioners had been in the area for generations and "…there's that sort of sense of belonging…" (Interview 9). It was perceived that some people had moved back to the area "because of family – they've got some kind of family connection here…" (Interview 4), again suggesting a sense of belonging. For others, the cheaper cost of housing has drawn people to the area or "…they came for work, or they came because they thought there may be work here but then there wasn't; so they've sort of ended up in the cheapest accommodation possible and putting up with conditions that aren't very nice" (Interview 4). It was also identified that there had been "an influx of minority groups coming to this area for farm work and cheap accommodation" (Interview 10) following the expansion of the EU.

The wellbeing aspects of living by the seaside were repeatedly commented on; for example, "…I think there are positive features because… you can breathe fresh air and there is lots of outdoor spaces that are generally pretty well maintained and kept" (Interview 9) and, in addition, it was "…perceived by people in London that it is a nicer place to be as it's near the seaside" (Interview 9). As Interview 9 continued "…if you're are looking at an old Victorian townhouse, even if you are only living in one room of it, from the outside it just looks much more appealing doesn't it, than a big tower block or a row of grey terraced that you might normally associate with deprivation."

Other features of the area were affirmed; for example, "I think there are loads of positive features, apart from the fact on a day like today with the sun shining, we've got beautiful beaches, clean beaches; there's a lot of regeneration work going on, the Turner gallery; the Turner Contemporary opens on the 16th April [2011] and that's bought with it regeneration in terms of arts and culture locally…" (Interview 1). National and international attention was focused on Margate when, on 11 November 2011, the Queen visited the Turner Contemporary gallery and promoted these positive aspects of Margate via the BBC. It is anticipated that this will attract an additional 135 000 visitors leading to an economic revival of the local economy.

Despite having many constructive influences on wellbeing identified, it was noted that for "…people that do have a lot of problems, it takes a long time for them to see the positives in the area…" (Interview 11). For example, "…you've got two, or three maybe, little boys living in a tiny little one-bedroom flat with no garden … you could just walk to the beach too, that doesn't necessarily occur to some people to do that" (Interview 9) and "I think for the families in this area, for a lot of them, the seaside is not necessarily an attraction for them; they're just dealing with the issues that they're dealing with… they're just dealing with the day-to-day aspects of living and the housing conditions" (Interview 7).

Community and family wellbeing – the contribution of the built environment

Many families are in private rented accommodation and it was identified that the population was quite mobile and transient "…sometimes they are waiting for social housing so they are maybe on a waiting list, or they've moved into the area temporarily" (Interview 7). This presents a range of challenges for promoting wellbeing when needs are identified; for example, "Families complaining about their housing conditions and not allowing us in to help them because that would affect their points in the housing register" (Interview 2). Many are also not registered with local services such as dentists and doctors, which has been identified through a local survey, *Your home, your health*. This reviews the health and wellbeing of individuals by doorstep questionnaires (Interview 2).

It was suggested that "Landlords seem to have become greedy. Where you possibly have five decent flats in the building, they would have ten, so obviously the knock-on effect of having a lot of people in a small area is the in-ing and out-ing, the banging, the noise, the arguments, and obviously you've got drug / mental health and alcohol problems in this area" (Interview 11). The detrimental impact of noise on psychological wellbeing is discussed by Habgood (2011) who identifies that an individual's response is personal, and thereby depends on not only the nature of the noise, but also its frequency, duration and timing. Habgood (2011) highlights that for legal action to be taken, it has to be deemed that the noise is a statutory nuisance, which is difficult to prove, making enforcement action challenging.

Sharing limited facilities within HMOs has a significant impact on the wellbeing of children and this was highlighted in an anonymous case study presented by Interviewee 9:

> "You've actually got to close the big gap of basic sort of personal hygiene because quite often if they come from poor housing they don't come to school clean or they haven't slept very well because they are sharing space with people that don't go to sleep till much later than them…you're having to address all these really quite basic needs before you can get the child on an even keel, before you can really start addressing higher order thinking skills which is really what schools are all about."

> "If you're in an overcrowded premises there's no space to do your homework; there's no space to actually flourish as a student." (Interview 1).

The issue of food poverty, associated with the shared living conditions and poor kitchen facilities, was highlighted in the interviews and has been the subject of other research in the Margate area, demonstrating the frequent difficulties HMO tenants face when attempting to prepare and eat a decent diet (Hopkins, 2011). Kayani (2009: 267) states that nutrition is important for wellbeing as it enhances the development of the brain, as well as being necessary for survival and is "intrinsic to emotional and mental security". Access to healthy food is not equitable either:

> "I think there are… massive issues to good quality cooking facilities, dietary issues for children and families living in the area… We know that many of them will opt to go and buy Pot Noodle rather than cooking on ancient or very poor, or virtually non-existent HMO facilities where a whole number of them are sharing one microwave" (Interview 1).

The difficulties for day-to-day family life were also highlighted:

> "If they have children, how can they have family orientation? They don't have a separate room to eat and sit down and chat with their children. It's all done on their knees because generally you have a room slightly bigger than this which is your kitchen and living room" (Interview 11).

One interviewee also commented, "We wondered about doing a survey of how many children had actually got a table in their house that they could sit at to do their homework" (Interview 9).

Safety within the home environment was highlighted on several occasions as an important wellbeing issue. Interviewee 4 commented "…I think it is realised more and more how much the effect of poor housing has on people and their general health and wellbeing. And I think for me my home is my haven. It's where you go at the end of the day and shut your door and shut the world out, and hopefully you feel safe and comfortable". (See also the discussion in *Chapter 5*).

For some interviewees this is not the reality of their experience:

> "…one child was reading a … book [at school] and it was called 'The Safe House', and what the book was about was things like don't leave your pan handle sticking out in the kitchen and stuff because … and don't have mats rucked up so you trip over; but the adult that was speaking to the child said 'Oh, what's safe about your house?' and the child said (it's a bit sad really)… 'You can hide under the kitchen table when the nasty people are outside'. Well at least you have a table I suppose" (Interview 9).

> "[The] building was taken over by a landlord and was investigated – I found that the actual property itself had an integral room which really wasn't particularly brilliant for fire safety and found a young family with a single baby living in a compartmented

room with no light. The only means of escape was out of the bedroom, so it was actually a room within a room basically" (Interview 6).

The findings presented here support the detrimental impact on family wellbeing and children's educational attainment as a result of deprivation, which is well documented.

APPROACHES TO ENHANCE FAMILY AND COMMUNITY WELLBEING

Taking on board the scope of wellbeing, there are many initiatives that have been undertaken by both statutory and non-statutory providers to tackle the unique issues facing family and community wellbeing in Margate. The Localism Act of 2011 has established the approach that should be used in regeneration projects and allows for national government policies to be applied while taking into account local circumstances, such as local markets, social profiles and local needs and aspirations. The Portas Review (Portas, 2011) ensured that Margate received £100 000 to boost local trade in the High Street.

The Margate Task Force, a multidisciplinary approach, sought to address the socio-economic disadvantages of these two wards. The Task Force Team comprises staff from a number of different organisations, including Thanet District Council, Kent County Council, Kent Police, Kent Fire and Rescue Service, Kent Probation, the Homes and Communities Agency, NHS Eastern and Coastal Kent, Jobcentre Plus and Connexions (Thanet District Council, 2011). The focus was on "housing regeneration, tackling low skills and worklessness, addressing health inequalities, reducing out of area placement of vulnerable people, and transforming the multi-agency delivery of services and community engagement" (Hill and Honey, 2010: 1). Aims include improving the quality of housing and the appearance of local neighbourhoods, preventing anti-social behaviour and providing improved support for residents who need it (Thanet District Council, 2011).

It was identified by interviewees that the Margate Task Force was a positive step forward; "…everyone recognises the problems like the deprivation we face in Cliftonville can't be faced by each individual service on its own… so the fact that we have integrated more of the public services that can contribute to the health and wellbeing agenda is all the better for us. Through the Margate Task Force we are getting a better picture of what people do…" (Interview 2), which is providing a "much more wrap-around service" (Interview 1).

Evidence of effective multidisciplinary team working in addressing specific family wellbeing needs was highlighted; for example:

"We had a family… they're quite a good example of a kind of a whole team working around that family; they were all in private rented housing, but each individual had an issue and there was drug use, alcohol use, children out of control, adolescents out of control, and children under the age of sort of twelve and thirteen and there were concerns of neglect. So what we had were there was police involvement, a community safety unit, Social Services. The younger children were on a child protect plan, educational welfare with the older children, and so a new professional approach was taken towards the family... the impact of all that work that was done... the family is stable..."(Interview 1).

Nevertheless, it was noted that this was the "beginning of a really good networking system... I think that there's a lot of work to do" (Interview 3) and that "...there are a lot of voluntary services that we are potentially unaware of at the moment that we need to tap into, and create those links between different groups" (Interview 3).

One of the main barriers to family and community wellbeing was felt to be a lack of social capital and social cohesion (i.e. the 'invisible glue' holding the community together, such as neighbourliness, trust and reciprocity) in the area. It is acknowledged that in areas where social capital is high, the level of crime is reduced, health outcomes are improved and there is higher educational attainment and improved income equality, with the subsequent effect of enhancing wellbeing (ONS, 2012). Social capital acquisition was felt to be a challenge locally because of the transient nature of the population. Several of those interviewed felt there was a need to promote social cohesion by being able to "introduce ways of stabilising the community for a period of time, so that we can get them into services to start with, so that we can help them to become more independent and that works for individuals and families" (Interview 3). Promoting owner occupation was felt to be an important way forward to establish social capital:

"We need to reduce the turn-around... we want a bit more of a family... try to reintroduce a bit more owner occupation... more commitment to the area, then obviously social capital will start to build and then obviously community pride... So better quality accommodation, keep providing the services that we can, mixed tenure, the more families, jobs... I mean mix it up... – if there's no jobs it's going to be difficult to mix it up" (Interview 2).

The Margate Task Force has sought to address, in particular, youth unemployment by developing apprenticeship opportunities with partnerships between Thanet District Council, Kent County Council and Thanet College (Thanet District Council, 2011).

The three Children's Centres within the area were identified as a positive feature to enhance family wellbeing. Children's Centres offer assistance to local families with children aged from birth up to sixteen years by providing information, advice and services. Interviewee 7 identified that these were places where:

"...parents can engage with their child(ren), ... you're learning with your child. They offer you different courses for that mum and the child develops well because it's Every Child Matters, so basically... and obviously the child gets used to being around children because again, when you're in a small confined space... it does have a knock-on effect for the mum, stressful for the mum, the mum is stressed out, the child feels it, so, you know… but life isn't simple, but you try and give them different things to go to" (Interview 11).

Despite measures to address the wellbeing of families in this seaside town, without a doubt services are overwhelmed and there are difficulties in recruiting social workers, teachers and health visitors to the area. For example:

"We become aware of a family living somewhere we think is having a detrimental impact on the wellbeing of the child, and if it's significant because there are an awful lot of children where we do think that it's [housing] having a detrimental impact but we know if we contact Social Services or whatever they'll say well actually loads of them are living like that, so if we think it is really bad and really significant then we make referrals to Social Services" (Interview 9).

CONCLUSION

Using the family and community context of wellbeing enables a useful perspective to consider many contemporary issues faced by those residents living in Margate, and indeed in seaside towns more generally. Such a context has enabled an initial exploration of challenges presented and an insight into good practice in this emerging agenda against a backdrop of growing poverty and inequality seemingly confounding efforts at supporting wellbeing at a local level.

It can be seen that within these two wards, there are a range of factors detrimentally affecting family and community wellbeing which perhaps are hidden behind the perception of the positive benefits of being beside the seaside. These factors have been highlighted locally and a range of initiatives introduced to enhance wellbeing. Much work has already been undertaken to develop and build upon existing networks and effective multidisciplinary team working, which is an important component in delivering the wellbeing agenda.

RESEARCH POINTER 8.1

- Identify a seaside town, either one you have visited or one you have found online. Explore what is being done there to enhance family and community wellbeing.

- What other initiatives could be implemented to enhance family and community wellbeing?

FURTHER READING

English Heritage and Urban Practitioners (2007) 'An Asset and a Challenge: Heritage and Regeneration in Coastal Towns in England': Final report. Available at: **www.helm.org.uk/guidance-library/asset-challenge-heritage-regeneration-coastal-towns-england/Coastal-Towns-Report3.pdf** [accessed 17 July 2013].

Knight, A. and McNaught, A. (Eds) (2011) *Understanding Wellbeing: An Introduction for Students and Practitioners of Health and Social Care*. Banbury: Lantern Publishing.

White, M., Smith, A., Humphryes, K., Pahl, S., Snelling, D., and Depledge, M. (2010) Blue Space: the importance of water for preference, affect and restorativeness ratings of natural and built scenes. *Journal of Environmental Psychology*, 30(4): 482–493.

09

GREEN SPACE AND WELLBEING

Nevin Mehmet and Christine Stacey

AIMS OF CHAPTER:

- To provide a background to why Green Spaces are crucial to Wellbeing;

- To explore the 'Grow Your Own Club', a community project to enhance community cohesion by developing the local physical environment;

- To apply the New Economic Foundation (NEF) (2008) 'Five Ways to Wellbeing' to develop synergy between people and the environment;

- To consider the relations between project-based activities and research.

INTRODUCTION

The current interest in, and focus on green spaces and community engagement has arisen from New Labour policy, specifically The Urban White Paper (DETR, 2000) on urban green spaces, that resulted in new funding opportunities, planning guidance, changes in urban green space governing and the introduction of national and local performance targets (Wilson and Hughes, 2011). The White Paper was the first Government initiative that focused on and evaluated how, why, or if exposure to green spaces impacts on psychological, emotional and spiritual health, and therefore wellbeing (Wilson and Hughes, 2011). The DETR (2000) paper aimed to limit urban sprawl by valuing the maintenance of green spaces, alongside the then Government's vision of urban areas, offering 'high quality of life' and 'opportunity for all'. What is interesting is that this has developed from the planning of new builds that incorporate public green areas, into the wider view that green space is a core concept for psychological health. With this has emerged a desire for a sustainable future (Wilson and Hughes, 2011) which includes greater participation in, for example, growing and sustaining our own food supply for people with space available to do so. Additionally, as Turner *et al*. (2010) argue, concern regarding how industrial agriculture has led to a disconnection between 'what we eat' and how 'food reaches our tables' has inspired projects where individuals can assume responsibility for what they eat.

With an increased population has come significant growth in urbanisation without green spaces. Research by Maas *et al.* (2006) highlights the positive association of people's perceived general health with green spaces. They play a vital role in the health and wellbeing of people, suggesting development and/or maintenance of green spaces be allocated a more central focus in planning policies. For instance, at national level in the UK, the Forestry Commission (2013) acknowledges the importance of integrating urban environments with green spaces, as this integration can be experienced as positive influences in promoting and enhancing health and wellbeing. Maas *et al.* (2006) also state that often people experience nature as an environment where they can "rest" and "recover" from the daily stress of an increasingly busy and pressurised lifestyle. Therefore, there is an increasing need for the availability of natural environments as a source of relaxation and recreation.

THE BACKDROP TO THE CULTIVATING LIVES PROJECT: ISLE OF SHEPPEY

The area of Swale is off the north coast of Kent in the Thames Estuary, approximately 46 miles east of London, consisting of three islands: Sheppey, Harty and Emley. The 'Cultivating Lives: Grow Your Own' (CLP) project took place on the Isle of Sheppey, which is approximately 36 square miles with a population of 37 000.

The Isle of Sheppey is separated from the mainland by the Swale Channel that enabled shipping to reach London's ports, avoiding the North Sea weather. In 1876, a large ferry terminal was built which included the Chatham and Dover Railway at Queensborough Pier, the naval dockyard, and commercial port. The steel industry formed a large part of the local economy, particularly for the dockyard workers. However, as ships became considerably larger, the decision was taken to close and transfer all work to Chatham in the late 1990s. This caused considerable economic dislocation for communities on Sheppey, resulting in limited employment opportunities, largely confined to the three prisons located on the island and the local tourist industry, bolstered by extensive and relatively unspoilt beaches.

Until 2006, a single lifting bridge provided access for everyone including train, pedestrians, bicycles and animals. To compound the isolation, public transport out of normal working hours is sparse, with buses stopping at 8 pm, and trains running only infrequently at night.

A new vehicular access bridge has been built. However, the closure of the passenger port has also significantly limited opportunities for growth and employment, creating further isolation of individuals and communities. Additionally, although there is a large supermarket on the island, fresh food costs are high due to the limited transport links. The retail industry is also sometimes reluctant to invest, because of the high levels of socio-economic deprivation in the area.

The Cultivating Lives Project (CLP) commenced in April 2009 and was one of several projects developed through the South East Coastal Communities (SECC) Project funded by the Higher Education Funding Council for England (HEFCE) to serve as demonstrator projects from 2008 to 2011. SECC's general goal was to promote collaborative work between nine universities in south-eastern England and their local communities, to enhance these communities' health and wellbeing.

The CLP arose from a Grow Your Own (food) Club (GYOC) developed initially by a local volunteer and an independent charitable trust, set up to support social and environmental regeneration through community engagement. The final project was developed between the local community and two local universities. The local Community Development Officer was actively involved in seeking the views of the local community, as to the ways and means that their community might be developed and improved. The project's main activities were ones based around sustainability, such as growing your own vegetables, and community-based regeneration/landscape activities, e.g. improving physical environment.

A Community Working Group sought views from the local community, through a variety of activities, including street interviews, community sessions and attendance at school open days. The decision was taken to develop the GYOC project into a scheme that would attract regeneration funding with the potential for significant impact. A consortium was therefore convened, and a bid prepared for SECC funding, which was approved in April 2009. The CLP was therefore designed to develop a sustainable environment, where the community could engage in useful and productive social and green activities. This would also provide a source of foodstuffs for the proposed community café in the community centre, alongside beautifying the local environment. In addition, it aimed to help develop, support and build local knowledge, capacity and skills; for example, the production of food and ornamental plants, shrubs and trees, and to ensure continued environmental sustainability.

WELLBEING IN PRACTICE
Community wellbeing – the contribution of the green environment

Allotments are often individual or communal plots of land to, for example, cultivate food or use for the recreational purpose of gardening. In the UK, allotments were associated more with the urban poor, who lived in crowded tenements, and were encouraged to grow their own (Wood *et al.*, 2012). These allotments have often been incorporated into new urban sprawl, and are now managed as collectives, which have seen the value of land rise, and are increasingly being sold off for building by private developers (National Allotment Society, 2013). This often means that their impact on wellbeing is ignored and not fully developed in terms of their contribution to urban environments. First and foremost, as social capital has declined in many areas, allotment schemes can help nurture new relationships, trust and reciprocal action, in communities across generations, gender and ethnic groups (Turner *et al.*, 2010), as well as being an important component of community and capacity development. At a time of increasing poverty and inequality, allotments can help provide local activities, cheaper foodstuffs and physical activity for the community. In short, they establish the 'missing link' from many area regeneration schemes and can provide a renewed focus around which the community can mobilise. For instance, the Eastside Roots Community Garden Centre in Bristol, which is a not-for-profit, volunteer-led cooperative, focused on promoting gardening, skills sharing and community building, has similar ideals and intentions as the CLP. Such schemes recognise that wellbeing cannot be compartmentalised, but involves various interfacing domains such as individuals, communities (Binley *et al.*, 2008) and the wider socio-economic/physical environment (La Placa *et al.*, 2013a; Knight and La Placa, 2013) which must be incorporated into research and practical-based projects intended to advance the role of wellbeing in public policy.

Urban environments are increasingly linear and individualised, often leading to isolation of individuals within the community, enabling researchers and community workers to develop the concept of 'community wellbeing' and its interactions with wider determinants (La Placa *et al.*, 2013b). However, according to Voicu and Been (2008), the issue of urban gardens, and the use of green space for recreation, is particularly contentious in cities, where there is pressure to sell off land for building homes that can then be sold at a profit. This creates tensions between those who view the physical environment as a community asset and those who see it as an economic windfall for urban development. Once this happens, whilst some members of cooperatives wish to retain the green spaces for the sake of the community, others see this as a form of commercial profit (Tranel and Handlin, 2006).

THE FIVE WAYS TO WELLBEING AS A FRAMEWORK FOR COMMUNITY PROJECTS

The UK Government Foresight Mental Capital and Wellbeing project's (2008) objective was to establish and address key issues that can impact on UK society over the following ten to twenty years, utilising evidence from a wide range of disciplines to analyse existing polices (Aked *et al.*, 2008). With the support of the Mental Capital and Wellbeing Project in 2008, the project analysed the most important drivers of psychological development and wellbeing to develop a long-term vision for psychological and social capital and wellbeing. From the evidence obtained, the centre for Wellbeing at the New Economics Foundation (NEF) was commissioned to develop evidence-based actions to improve personal, social and economic wellbeing. Within the initial phase, NEF (2008) utilised the long list of actions for enhancing wellbeing based on the Foresight Programme (2008) and emerging literature in positive psychology. The NEF was given the challenge of creating an approach that was innovative in design, and would be widely used to promote and support the improvement of wellbeing in a way that reflected the key findings within current research.

A set of five key messages on the evidence around 'social relationships', 'physical activity', 'awareness', 'learning' and 'giving' was created to effectively communicate the main influencers of wellbeing (NEF, 2008). These messages have been organised into five key actions that offer examples of more specific behaviour that enhances wellbeing. The Five

Ways to Wellbeing are 'Connect', 'Be active', 'Take Notice', 'Keep Learning' and 'Give' (NEF, 2008). The Five Ways to Wellbeing are used by health organisations, schools and community projects across the UK, and globally, as a framework to support individuals in improving their wellbeing, via organisational strategies to measure impact, assess need and encourage communities and individuals to incorporate wellbeing activities into their environments and lives (NEF, 2008).

In the context of the CLP, the application of the Five Ways to Wellbeing provides a contextualised approach, highlighting the way in which this strategy can be applied to support a community's wellbeing needs. Beginning with the NEF's (2008) 'Connect', one of the key outcomes of the CLP, was to establish a more connected and driven community, for sustainable community growth. Connect is viewed by Aked *et al.* (2008) as the cornerstone of individuals' and communities' lived experiences, by building sustainable connections to support and enrich their lives. The CLP aimed to build a stronger community, by encouraging individuals within the community to work together with stakeholders, to support social and environmental regeneration, through community engagement. This is supported by the Foresight Report (2008) that indicated how social relationships are critical in promoting wellbeing and supporting mental health across all ages. One example was the 'Going Potty' event whereby members from the local community, students from the local school, and individuals from the local day centre for people with learning disabilities, were brought together to make hanging baskets that could be used to beautify the Community Centre. One of the positive aspects of the CLP was that these activities and events brought the community together, while encouraging regeneration of the area. This is supported by Morrow (2001) who reminds us of the significance of social capital, in particular the development of social networks, to promote a sense of belonging to a community, which will in turn enhance wellbeing (La Placa *et al.*, 2013a).

The CLP relied heavily on the community to engage physically in the regeneration and beautification of the area, which supports 'Be Active', as a way to wellbeing. Kirkwood *et al.* (2008) report that engagement in physical activity is considered beneficial to wellbeing by increasing perceived self-efficacy, a sense of mastery and a perceived ability to cope. The whole project was based on the idea of the community maintaining a level of activity within gardening and horticultural activities. For example, the clearance of land space, surrounding the project, was undertaken by young people from the Future Jobs Fund. Physical activity such as gardening (Clatworthy, 2012) was incorporated into encouraging social interactions and enhancing wellbeing.

The third aspect of the NEF (2008), 'Take Notice', encourages individuals to develop self-awareness of their surroundings and identification with the community. Aked *et al.* (2008) argue that such activities can encourage either a behaviour change or a change in the environment, which can in turn precipitate positive behaviour. For example, the head of a local school invited pupils at risk of school exclusion to undertake a variety of simple tasks that included painting and decorating activities, with the outcome that their behaviour improved and risk of school exclusion was reduced. The 'clean up' stage of the project further supported individuals to identify the immediate environment that required beautification or regeneration. This resulted in the successful application for a further grant that gave rise to more community activities around tree planting, culminating in the planting of 500 whip trees, to enhance what was considered an unkempt area. The area around the newly converted community centre, and along the adjacent kerbside, was also planted with hundreds of annual flowering shrubs. It was intended that such beautification would encourage a sense of community ownership and the need for a sustainable environment.

Aked *et al.* (2008) assert that by being mindful (the state of being attentive to and aware of what is occurring in present circumstances) has also been shown to predict positive psychological health and heightened self-knowledge, which can support the fourth way to wellbeing, 'Keep Learning'. Adult learning has been correlated with positive effects on wellbeing and social interaction (Aked *et al.*, 2008). A key element of the project's outcome was increased education and knowledge of horticulture and agriculture; for example, the creation of small business enterprise volunteers, to learn to cultivate their own fruit and vegetables. The teaching and knowledge was supplied by a local charity and resulted in enough produce being provided to enable the community centre to sell inexpensive but nourishing meals. As Hammond (2004) highlights, common goals not only lead to satisfaction and development within the community, but also provide a positive impact in individual growth and personal wellbeing.

Lastly, 'Give' is the fifth strategy in maximising wellbeing and incorporates the "doing of something nice and/or supportive for a friend, neighbour or stranger or by supporting the local community" and developing reciprocal relations. The Foresight project (2008) found active participation in social and community life, particularly volunteering, provides purpose and meaning for participants. The GYOC club within the project was a fundamental component of the whole process, where volunteers supported the cultivation of the vegetables and fruit within the community garden. The produce was then cooked by offenders from the local open prison under supervision of the café, providing inexpensive but nutritious meals in a warm environment, where people who were socially isolated and economically deprived could come and receive a meal. The other aspect was that the offenders learnt skills which they could transfer to future employment opportunities, and reduce the risk of reoffending. The café was kept open by volunteers from the community to support the day-to-day running of the café. The café soon became the 'hub' of the community, whereby individuals developed a sense of contributing to the community. The profits from the café were returned to support the development of the produce. This activity alone comprehensively incorporated the five ways to wellbeing and demonstrated how a simply designed project idea could become a model for change and develop a co-productive approach (Knight and La Placa, 2013).

EVALUATION OF THE PROJECT

As previously mentioned, the main objective of the CLP (2009) project was to help develop, support and build the fledgling 'Grow Your Own' Club, by partnering with other organisations to build knowledge, capacity and skills in, for instance, the production of food and ornamental plants, shrubs and trees, to ensure continued environmental sustainability. When the project was formally evaluated, through a range of quantitative and qualitative consultation methods, the most noticeable finding was the requirement to have experienced project managers, and the need to design projects within available funding. As Haponava and Al-Jibouri (2012) have identified, project management involves reflection, learning and experience as well as practical ability.

Capacity to involve and consult others requires a reflective perspective, which can often be absent when the day-to-day practical skills of implementation and organisation seem paramount. However, in terms of enhancing community participation, evaluation demonstrated that participants felt connected to the project, an important component of the 'Connect' aspect of the Five Ways to Wellbeing. The evaluation also found that stakeholder consultation with service users and designers should have been more interactive throughout the time span of the project, enabling the ongoing revision of aims and objectives, based upon participants' perspectives. However, overall, the evaluation concluded that integration of people into the physical and geographical locality not only enhanced the physical environment, but gave individuals a sense of purpose, community integration, ownership of the environment and enhancement of wellbeing. The project fulfilled the application of the Five Ways to Wellbeing and provided a useful example of how the physical, personal and social domains of wellbeing interacted (La Placa *et al.*, 2013a). Individuals did indeed develop enhanced relationships and self-awareness, and feel a sense of purpose and contribution to activities that improve the environment. If volunteerism is to be made attractive in communities, we believe those involved need to reflect and develop the ability to react to ever-changing requirements and employ the Five Ways to Wellbeing to assess success. We now turn to issues of project-based activities and research processes.

PROJECT-BASED ACTIVITIES AND RESEARCH

Although this was not intended to be a research project, significant lessons were learned about communities and their development, when approached as a case study. Peel *et al.* (2010) demonstrated how evidence can be accumulated from an intervention as a process development, and the experience of implementing a project can produce evidence for further design and revision. Informal and local projects are similar to formal research evaluations too, in that they require similar strategy, knowledge and practical skills to more formal research (Stoecker, 2013). For instance, 'project' definition and risk management, seeking funding, the writing of funding bids, developing and leading the project team, the instigation and management of the project, monitoring and control, evaluation and identification of lessons learned, mirror many of the aspects of the formal 'research' project and/or evaluation of an intervention.

Therefore local project work can be considered an effective training ground for individuals who might want to become involved in further research and evaluation. Researchers can often experience difficulties with sampling and researching vulnerable groups, but individuals concerned with developing projects (involving such people) can often dissolve the barriers by the very process of providing a service and enhancing participation (Stoecker, 2013). Project design and implementation can be used to bridge power imbalances between researchers and marginalised communities (Dharamsi *et al.*, 2010). The concept of community action is relevant here, whereby service users, communities and community developers coalesce to design research questions, and involve the community in solutions (Knight and La Placa, 2013). This is similar to the arguments made by La Placa *et al.* in this book's conclusion, that wellbeing interventions be made relevant to professional and lay people alike.

Whitney *et al.* (2009) and Struyk and Haddaway (2011) have also highlighted the synergy between project development and research strategies in the social sciences. Practical knowledge in the form of devising and implementing projects can be a source of evidence, very much like formal research, conducted by experienced researchers and policy makers. This is particularly the case with community development initiatives that stress involvement and the 'bottom up' approach, as opposed to traditional community-based health improvement work. The latter is more inclined to be 'top down' and professional and agency driven (Cowie and Mages, 2011). Nevertheless, we believe this does not remove the need for lay people involved in project work to be consulted by experienced researchers in evaluations of their services, if they reflect their lived experiences, and are used to facilitate more effective design of services and good governance. In fact, lived experience is a process that should be included in both project-based and formal research-based work. Both can aim at service improvement and community development and can be predicated upon social justice (Whitmore *et al.*, 2013). Researchers and communities alike can facilitate changes in the environment and the use of services. For example, groups and individuals involved in the service or initiative should, we think, be included in design of methodologies to evaluate them. Evaluators and professionals, on the other hand, can incorporate capacity to advise on new ways of bringing communities together and delivering community services, based on those they researched.

CONCLUSION

This chapter has provided a background as to why green spaces are crucial to wellbeing and explored the use of an environmental community project to develop and enhance community cohesion and wellbeing. It has applied the NEF's (2008) 'Five Ways to Wellbeing' to develop synergy between people and their environment, and briefly considered how the practical implementation of project-based community activities can be as effective as research-based activities to policy makers and community developers. It has provided an illustration of the physical environment as one domain of wellbeing among others, and illustrated evidence of utilising the physical environment to enhance aspects of wellbeing and community cohesion.

RESEARCH POINTER 9.1

Identify an urban area that you think could be beautified.

- Explore what you think could be done to enhance the area for community wellbeing.

- What other initiatives could be implemented to enhance community wellbeing?

- Using the tool outlined below, how would you develop your project?

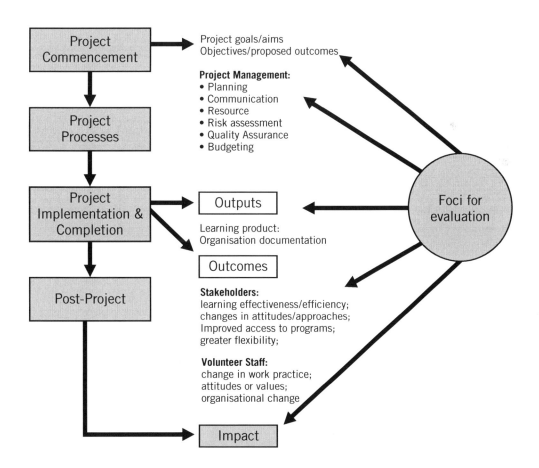

FURTHER READING

Harvey, J. and Taylor, V. (2013) *Measuring Health and Wellbeing*. London: Sage.

Stoecker, R. (2013) *Research Methods for Community Change: a Project-Based Approach* 2nd edn. London: Sage.

Taylor, G. and Hawley, H. (2010) *Key Debates in Health Care*. Maidenhead: Open University Press, McGraw-Hill.

10

A GLOBAL GLIMPSE: WELLBEING AND ISLAM

Allan McNaught

AIMS OF CHAPTER:

- To identify and examine Islamic concepts of wellbeing and contrast these with Western concepts of wellbeing;

- To debate the implications of our understanding of wellbeing by religion;

- To review and contextualise studies that operationalise Islamic concepts of wellbeing for individuals, families, communities and societies more broadly;

- To explore the implications on assessing and measuring wellbeing among Muslims using Western designed research tools.

INTRODUCTION

There is a considerable body of research, debate and thinking on wellbeing, and much of this is reflected in the Islamic world. This chapter will explore the influence of the Islamic faith on individual, family, community and societal wellbeing, drawing on the available research evidence. It will be a theoretical and conceptual discussion to give an appreciation of the scope of the field of study. The exploration was based on a number of research questions, but no hypothesis. Using my own definitional framework as a guide, my key question is "What does wellbeing mean in Islam?" Subsidiary questions include: does the application of Islamic principles and values result in a very different construction of wellbeing from others in use? How is this construct measured, if it exists? What other factors and domains need to be accounted for in constructing an Islamic definition of wellbeing, given that religious processes often interact with other global ones? I have written previously on the theme of developing a framework for defining wellbeing that is more inclusive, and reflects the complexity of the individual's social existence, and which incorporates objective as well as subjective assessment (McNaught, 2011; La Placa *et al.*, 2013a). This framework is depicted in *Figure 10.1*. It identifies four interacting domains of wellbeing: individual; family; community and society, which are comprised

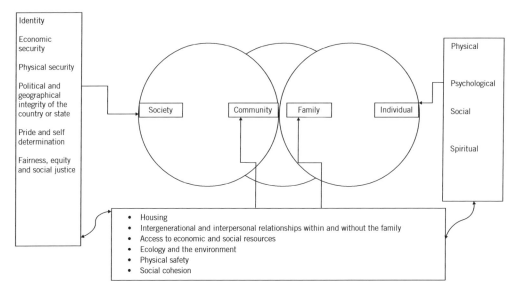

Figure 10.1 *Framework for defining wellbeing.*
Source: McNaught (2011).

of various sub-categories of processes and relations. This enables objective and subjective assessments of the domains.

This chapter will use this framework as a guide to explore the meaning of wellbeing to followers of Islam. This will be of necessity a limited exploration, but one which I hope will highlight the thinking, as well as the application of wellbeing theories and measurement instruments to Muslim populations.

UNDERSTANDING ISLAM

Islam is an Arabic word meaning 'submission, surrender, and obedience'. Islam stands for complete submission and obedience to Allah (God) (Ahmad, 1959). The adherents to Islam are called Muslims. The UK Muslim populations are from varied sources, including Arabs and Turks from the Middle East and North Africa (the MENA region), as well as Muslims from West Africa, Pakistan and Bangladesh. There are also an unknown number of British and European people who have converted to Islam (Suleiman, 2013). Worldwide, the largest concentration of Muslims is in South East Asia (Indonesia and Malaysia). There are also large Muslim populations in West and East Africa, the former Soviet Republics in Central Asia (Uzbekistan, Kazakhstan, Kyrgyzstan, Turkmenistan) as well as in India, Pakistan, and Bosnia and Herzegovina. For a geographic distribution of the World's Muslim populations, see **http://graphtheworld.blogspot.ae/2012/01/map-muslim-population-in-world.html**

There are some states that are officially called Islamic Republics (Iran, Afghanistan, and Pakistan), and some Muslim majority countries (MMC), such as Indonesia, the Maldives and Malaysia. Apart from the three Islamic Republics mentioned previously, only the Kingdom of Saudi Arabia has legal systems based wholly on Islamic (Sharia) law. There are some other countries that have mixed legal systems, of which Sharia is one part. There are conflicts in some states over some regions or groups attempting to apply Sharia law in their area, in violation of the constitution, and against the wishes of the majority population (Nigeria, Mali and Indonesia).

It is important to understand the scope and impact of Islam on people's day-to-day lives. Hamidi and Jadiry (1979) note that "In addition to being a religious book (the Quran), it also covers legal, social, educative and humanitarian codes that had provided the Islamic nation with all the sound principles for the development of their community. It may be viewed as a comprehensive encyclopedia to serve humanity in every (aspect) of life" (ibid., 1979). The main tenets of the religion are detailed in the remainder of this section:

Belief in God

Muslims believe in one God, who has neither son nor partner, and that none has the right to be worshipped, but him alone. In the Quran, God is described in the following way: "He is God, the One; God, to whom the creatures turn for their needs. He begets not, nor was He begotten, and there is none like Him" (Quran, 2004: Chapter 112: 1–4).

Belief in the angels

Muslims believe in the existence of the angels and that they are honoured creatures. The angels worship God alone, obey him, and act only by his command. Among the angels is Gabriel, who is the messenger that communicated the Quran from God to Prophet Muhammad.

Belief in God's revealed books

Muslims believe that God revealed books to his messengers as proof for mankind and as guidance for them. Among these books is the Quran. God has guaranteed the Quran's protection from any corruption or distortion; "Indeed, we have sent down the Quran, and surely we will guard it [from corruption] (Quran, 2004: 15: 9).

Belief in the prophets and messengers of God

Muslims believe in the prophets and messengers of God, starting with Adam and including Noah, Abraham, Ishmael, Isaac, Jacob, Moses, and Jesus. But God's final message to man, a reconfirmation of the eternal message, was revealed to the Prophet Muhammad. Muslims believe that Muhammad is the last prophet sent by God: "Muhammad is not the father of any one of your men, but he is the Messenger of God and the last of the prophets" (Quran, 20004: 33: 40).

Belief in the Day of Judgment

Muslims believe in the Day of Judgment (the Day of Resurrection) when all people will be resurrected for God's judgment according to their beliefs and deeds.

Belief in faith

Muslims believe in Al-Qadar, which is divine predestination, a belief that God is all-knowing and wills events; this belief does not discount exercise of free will. Muslims believe we can choose right or wrong and that we are responsible for our choices.

The Five Pillars of Islam

The Five Pillars of Islam are the framework of Islamic life. They are:

1. The testimony of faith (Shahada) that there is only one God and Muhammad is the Messenger of faith
2. Prayer, a direct link between the worshipper and God
3. Giving Zakat (support of the poor and needy)
4. Fasting during the month of Ramadan to gain enriched spiritual knowledge, awareness and self-purification
5. Pilgrimage to Makkah once in a lifetime for those who are able. It is here that forgiveness is sought and is often thought of as a preview of the 'Day of Judgment'.

RELIGIOUS OBSERVANCE AND WELLBEING

There is a considerable volume of Islamic literature on the topic of 'happiness' (Al-Ghazzali, 1910; Mihr, 1990; Masir and Adam, 1995). This genre of work is aimed at practising Muslims and seems to offer spiritual guidance and to further bolster them in their faith. For example, Shahran (2009) observes that in the Quran, happiness is described by the word *sa'adah*. Whenever the term *sa'adah* is mentioned in the Quran, it is always related to two conditions: the happiness in the hereafter (*ukhrawiyyah*) and happiness in the present world. For a Muslim, the ultimate happiness is that of the hereafter, as mentioned by the Almighty Allah in Surah Hud (Shahran, 2009) as well as ability to do all God has commanded.

This literature is very much a debate within Islam. However, there have been instances when this debate has crossed over and challenged mainstream subjective wellbeing/"happiness theories" (Moosavi, 2005; 2006a; 2006b; 2008). "Obtaining authentic happiness depends on faith and moral acts… a purified and exalted life is at a level higher than normal and primitive life… authentic happiness means attaining a purified or comprehensive life which is filled with meaning and purpose" (Moosavi, 2006b: 4). One can see why Islamic scholars might take issue with the constructs of subjective wellbeing advanced by psychologists, as there is a fundamental philosophical divide between the two ways of thinking about wellbeing. The

Islamic approach seems to be around conforming to Islamic values and principles and their behavioural corollaries, meaning that the Islamic construct of wellbeing has stronger moral and theological components than is the norm in a Western conceptualisation of wellbeing.

The wellbeing of individuals and populations can be assessed subjectively and objectively (Woodlock, 2012). While there is a considerable body of research on religion, health and wellbeing, surprisingly little of it focuses specifically on Islam and wellbeing, either subjectively or objectively. The prevailing literature attempts to explore the correlation between religious observance, wellbeing and health (Kaldor *et al.*, 2004; Caras, 2003; Steiner *et al.*, 2010). Much of this literature is concerned with Christianity, and tries to relate measures of health and wellbeing to proxies for the strength or frequency of religious practice. With Islam and wellbeing, we have a more complex phenomenon, in that Islam is a way of life, and is far more integral to a person's existence and routines than with other religions. Another complexity with the focus on Islam is that the religion has devotees in many cultural, ethnic and national groups, and their practice of Islam has been integrated with pre-existing cultures and traditions.

It has been long established that there is a link between religion / spirituality and wellbeing, and this seems to hold across all faith groups (Knight and Khan, 2011; Fredrickson, 2002). My own 'structured framework for defining wellbeing' (McNaught, 2011) recognises spirituality as an integral components of individual wellbeing. Given the influence of Islam on its followers, it would be reasonable to also include religion / spirituality as a factor in family, community and societal wellbeing.

There is a lack of clarity about the precise processes or mechanisms through which religion produces the wellbeing effect. It is frequently assumed that it is the positive emotions associated with religion that explains the benefit of religion on wellbeing. Kaldor *et al.* (2004) explored the extent to which willingness to develop one's spirituality related to higher levels of wellbeing. They found that there was a positive relationship between religious beliefs and active involvement in private or public religious practice, and many of the measures of wellbeing. The analysis of the data suggests that those with more orthodox religious belief tend to record higher levels of optimism, a sense of purpose in life, and involvement in caring activities.

MEASURING SUBJECTIVE WELLBEING WITHIN MUSLIM POPULATIONS

There are a number of studies that attempt to measure the subjective wellbeing of Muslim populations, either exclusively, or by including some Muslim respondents in their survey sample. Aflakseir (2012) has explored the relationship between "the sense of personal meaning, psychological wellbeing, spirituality and religiosity" of a group of Muslim students in England. His hypothesis was that there would be a positive relationship between personal meanings, psychological wellbeing, and spirituality and religiosity. Sixty respondents were recruited at universities in Birmingham and Southampton; four research instruments were used to assess their wellbeing. These were: The Life Attitude Profile Revised, the Sources of Meaning Profile – Revised Scale, The Psychological Wellbeing Scale and the Strength of Spiritual Belief Scale.

The findings were that Muslim students who practised their religion perceived their life as meaningful. The researcher noted some other differences in this cohort with other population groups. These differences related to Death Acceptance and Choice/Responsibility, which were the two components of the questionnaire used to assess wellbeing. These differences were attributed to conflict with Islamic teaching/philosophy. He speculates that "religion enhances meaning of life by providing a unifying philosophy of life and serves as an integrating and stabilizing force that provides a framework for interpreting life's challenges and provides a resolution to difficult conditions" (ibid.: 30).

Wan Ibrahim *et al.* (2012) have reported a study of subjective wellbeing of older Muslims in rural areas of Malaysia. This was a very conventional study in which the population seems to have been selected more for their demographic characteristics, as there was no focus on any aspect of their faith in either the methodology or the reported findings.

A significant body of research has been conducted in Kuwait by Abdel-Khalek (Abdel-Khalek, 2004, 2006a, 2008 and 2010). This work consists largely of quality of life measurement. One study in particular (2006a) attempts to test the link "between, and gender differences in, happiness, physical health, mental health and religiosity" (ibid.: 85). This study included a relatively large sample of 2210 male and 1154 female undergraduates. Four self-rating scales were used to assess happiness, physical health, mental health and religiosity.

The main finding of the study is the "significant relation between the self-ratings of happiness, physical health, mental health and religiosity (ibid.: 93), and it is noted "religion is more central and plays a more important role in Kuwaiti society" (ibid.: 93). These findings were confirmed in a later study of 424 adult employees (Abdel-Khalek, 2008), and in a sample of 224 Egyptian college students (Abdel-Khalek, 2010).

This link between religiosity and happiness has produced contrary findings among Christians (Lewis, 2002: Lewis *et al.*, 1997). Indeed, it could be argued that the patterns of devotion and religious observance among Christians, Muslims and other religious communities can vary in intensity. In addition, Islam extends beyond religious practices, and shapes the adherent's day-to-day life, and the structure of their existence. As such, any comparative research therefore needs to include more complex measures beyond the extent of religious practice, if we are to be assured that we are comparing similar phenomena. Another weakness of these studies of happiness and subjective and psychological wellbeing is that they deal with internal states and do not move beyond the individual to assess the social, cultural and environmental drivers of wellbeing.

An example is the findings of Moghnie and Kazarian's (2012) evaluation of the subjective wellbeing of college students in Lebanon. The instrument was an Arabic translation of the Subjective Happiness Scale (SHS) and the Parental Acceptance Questionnaire (PARQ), administered to 273 students in state and private colleges. This study does not objectively take religion into account, and is more concerned with the reliability and cultural appropriateness of the measuring instrument. The subjective happiness scores of Lebanese students were below those of US college students. This is not surprising, given that they are challenged by waves of economic and political instability that undermine their employment opportunities and contribute to their migration to other countries for economic livelihood and stability.

The impact of environmental factors on assessing the influence of religiosity and spirituality on wellbeing was noted by Tiliouine *et al.* (2009) in their study of Islamic wellbeing in Algeria. In their study of 2909 Muslims, religiosity was found not to contribute towards wellbeing as they measured it. It was postulated that the post-conflict situation in the country and reassumption of normal life were the major concerns of respondents.

Woodlock (2012) studied the subjective and national wellbeing of a sample of Muslims in comparison with the general population in two regions in Australia. There were 600 people in the sample for a questionnaire-based survey. Subjective wellbeing referred to how individuals perceive their life circumstances. National wellbeing is not defined, but it seems to refer to the wellbeing of Muslims as a distinct community. The survey found that in respect of personal wellbeing, Muslim scores were indistinguishable from those of the general Australian population. However, there were differences in two domains: those of safety and future security. It was hypothesised by Cummins *et al.* (2003), cited in Woodlock (2012), that Muslims might feel vulnerable due to "world crisis" events involving Muslims elsewhere. The local corollary of these events is increased scrutiny, anti-Muslim political rhetoric, and racial and religious vilification. With national wellbeing, Muslims fare worse than the rest of Australia's populations, with significantly less satisfaction over the role of government than the general population. Again it is hypothesised that this finding could arise from the "positioning of Muslims as a potential threat" (ibid.: 197).

The studies that have been summarised so far suggest that while it is possible for Muslims and other individuals to experience high subjective wellbeing, their wellbeing can be compromised at other levels and locations within their social system, over which they have no control. In the extreme, these 'extraneous' forces might prove an existential threat to the individual or the community concerned. The political and social rhetoric surrounding the global war on terror has provided fertile breeding ground for anti-Muslim, right wing politics in many countries. The social pressures resulting from the austerity programmes that have followed the financial crisis have heightened anti-immigrant and anti-Muslim sentiments in many countries.

Within the UK, Muslims have long been a disadvantaged group. According to Laird *et al.* (2007), when compared to other religious groups, Muslims in the UK have the highest age-standardised rate of reported ill health (13% for males, 16% for females) and disability (24% of females, 21% of males), with widespread poverty and deprivation. Muslims in the USA generally have higher socio-economic status than their UK counterparts, although the range is wide. Specific health research data are sparse, and information on Muslim youth even more limited.

Much of the focus in the UK is on Muslims as an ethnic group and a perceived security threat; however, this also masks the significant religious discrimination that they experience, because discrimination is often expressed as being against cultural practices, as opposed to their religious practices and beliefs. Laird *et al.* (2007) cite the identification by Weller *et al.* (2001) of six levels of religious discrimination, all of which are pertinent to the day-to-day life of Muslims in the UK. Muslims in Western societies experience a patchwork of ethical/racial and religious discrimination; overlaid onto this is the antipathy, antagonism and violence directed towards Muslim communities, who may be perceived to be allied with terrorists or instigators of terrorism.

FAMILY AND COMMUNITY WELLBEING

My literature search only discovered one study that focused on household or family wellbeing in Malaysia (Abdelhak and Sulaiman, 2001). This study focused on household wellbeing, poverty alleviation and the role played by Islamic values. It also explored the use and role of Islamic vehicles for the support of the poor: Zakat, Sadakah (see below) and interest-free loans. It sought to shed light on the underlying gap between Islamic values and principles that could substantially enhance people's wellbeing and alleviate their vulnerability to poverty (ibid.: 3). In the context of household poverty, the researchers were concerned with two questions, as follows:

1. How do Islamic values and principles contribute to people's wellbeing?
2. Do these values and principles serve positively or otherwise in helping to prevent households falling into poverty traps? (ibid.: 3).

The Islamic expectation is that individuals should work to support themselves and their family, and that family finances should be managed effectively. It is also the person's duty to enhance his or her skills and talents to enhance work and productivity. Community responsibility takes the shape of Zakat, Sadakah and Waqf, and interest-free loans. Zakat is compulsory, and is a way of sharing wealth. Sadakah and Waqf are charitable donation and activities, and Muslims are encouraged to be involved in these matters, as an act of piety and goodness. Government obligations take the shape of transfer payments, facilitating economic growth, and measures for equal opportunities.

Data were collected via a structured socio-economic questionnaire containing open- and closed-ended questions. After piloting the questionnaire on 30 people, a final sample of

100 respondents was selected. All respondents had received or had been involved in some type of Islamic scheme, such as Zakat, Sadakah or an interest-free loan. Following the questionnaire, individuals were further assessed to measure the impact of Islamic values and principles on household wellbeing and their contribution to avoidance of poverty traps. The results suggested that the degree of an individual's self-responsibility was "a fundamental key in eradicating his own poverty" (ibid.: 14). Those individuals who succeeded were characterised by self-belief, optimism, frequent prayer and a self-improvement ethos. These individuals were more likely to seek interest-free loans, as opposed to support from Zakat/Sadakah (charity).

Households that had received Zakat/Sadakah were poorer, less optimistic and less orientated towards self-improvement. The study concluded that motivation was the key to poverty alleviation, and that those households that were more successful in managing their circumstances were those that adhered to Islamic values and principles. The researchers recommended that charitable support should be provided through the Islamic financial system (i.e. interest-free loans, as opposed to charity) to improve the motivation of the poor.

SOCIETAL WELLBEING: AN ISLAMIC DIMENSION

If we focus on MMC, how should wellbeing be measured and what is the evidence about the wellbeing of individuals or communities? The studies quoted from Kuwait, Lebanon and Malaysia proceed some way to providing answers. In addition we can look at the available evidence/measures at societal or national level. Two distinct approaches to societal and national wellbeing have emerged. One is anchored in the concept of 'happiness', and indices have been developed to measure happiness (Helliwell et al., 2013). The other focuses on development, using such measure as the Human Development Index (HDI), which is reported upon annually by the United Nations Development Programme (UNDP, 2013). The HDI is used as a measure to rank countries by their level of development. The general assumption is that the higher the HDI, the higher the level of wellbeing experienced by the residents of the countries concerned. The 2011 ranking for MMC is shown in *Table 10.1*.

Whilst it could be argued that the HDI does measure certain aspects of human development, it is not designed to reflect the nuances and workings of a society organised on religious principles. Hendrie Anto (2009) has argued that the Islamic perspective on economic development is different from conventional perspectives in that it emphasises comprehensive and holistic welfare in this world and hereafter (Falah). The existing HDI published by UNDP might be the most comprehensive indicator (of human development), but it is not fully compatible and sufficient for measuring human development in an Islamic perspective.

The author proceeds to develop an Islamic Human Development Index (IHDI). This new measure is considered within the framework of Maqasid *al-Shari'ah*, which is concerned with

Table 10.1 *2011 Human Development Index ranking for Muslim Majority Countries*

VERY HIGH HDI		Azerbaijan	0.734	Indonesia	0.629
Brunei	0.855	Oman	0.731	Maldives	0.688
Qatar	0.834	Turkey	0.722	Kyrgyzstan	0.622
UAE	0.818	Algeria	0.713	Tajikistan	0.622
HIGH HDI		Tunisia	0.712	Morocco	0.582
Bahrain	0.796	MEDIUM HDI		LOW HDI	
Kuwait	0.790	Jordan	0.700	Pakistan	0.515
Saudi Arabia	0.782	Algeria	0.700	Bangladesh	0.515
Malaysia	0.769	Turkmenistan	0.698	Yemen	0.458
Kazakhstan	0.754	Egypt	0.622	Senegal	0.470
Iran	0.742	Palestine	0.641	Mauritania	0.467
Lebanon	0.745	Uzbekistan	0.641	Djibouti	0.445
Libya	0.769	Syria	0.632	Afghanistan	0.374

Source: UNDP (2013) Human Development Report.

the promotion of human wellbeing, through the preservation of self, wealth, posterity, intellect and faith (Hendrie Anto, 2009). This reformulation results in seven additional indices. The IHDI is then constructed and used to assess countries in a league table. The outcome is a slight difference in the ranking, with some countries faring better on this new index as compared with the HDI. Some countries experience a marked deterioration in rank. However, the countries at the top and bottom remain largely the same, although ranked differently.

As an extension of this approach, Batchelor (2006) has developed an Islamic Index of Wellbeing, based on the Quran and the Sunnah. The key indices are religiosity (the percentage of Muslims who perform the obligatory prayers five times daily, men attending mosque at least once per week, fasting for Ramadan and paying Zakat) and what is termed "social interactions" (levels of secondary education, status of women, care of children, and the poor).

Indices were calculated for 27 of the 50 MMC, plus Nigeria. The Gulf States were not included in the survey. The results ranked Malaysia and Indonesia in the top two positions, followed by Senegal, and the Palestine Territories. In the next band are MENA countries and then sub-Saharan Africa, which overlap. The former communist bloc countries generally had the lowest indices on this calculation.

The measurement of happiness has been a concern for the past decade, stimulated by developments in happiness measurement in Bhutan, Canada, France, and, more recently, the UK. In July 2011, the United Nations General Assembly passed a resolution inviting member countries to measure the happiness of their people and to use this to help guide their public policies. An independent group of experts has now produced two annual World Happiness Reports (Helliwell *et al.*, 2012; 2013). In the 2013 report, Sachs (2013) argues for a return to virtue ethics in the pursuit of happiness. In so doing, he compares the values of Buddhism, virtue ethics and Christianity as paths to happiness as compared with consumerism/materialism.

CONCLUSION

Happiness and wellbeing are a major concern in Islam, reflected in a body of publications, which explore the meaning of happiness in Islam. I cannot say if the works that I have quoted are representative, but happiness in Islam seems to have a stronger moral and philosophical core than in Western discourse. This is not surprising, given the role of religion in society (Lee and Newburg, 2005). However, I could not find any evidence that an Islamic concept of wellbeing has been operationalised and measured on an individual level.

There are numerous examples of Western-derived subjective wellbeing SWB assessment being undertaken on Muslim individuals and communities in the West, South Asia and the Middle East. Given the internal logic of the instruments used, the results are not surprising. The shortcomings of these measures are demonstrated in the research in Lebanon, whereby high levels of SWB are influenced by high levels of national instability and personal disruption. This result is confirmation of Woodlock's observation that "Personal wellbeing is held under homeostatic control and supported by external factors and internal factors" (Woodlock, 2012: 126). My literature search only discovered one study that focused on household or family wellbeing (Abdelhak and Sulaiman, 2001). The emphasis on self-responsibility and charity as core Islamic values and principles was a striking feature of this work, along with a clear expression of community (brotherhood) and governmental responsibility. This conveys a more sober and less 'self-obsessed' view of wellbeing than is prevalent in Western culture.

This is also reflected at a community level, where Zakat, Sadakah and Waqf, and interest-free loans are the main forms of assistance to others, and these seem to be more important than social security or other forms of state aid. These acts, and the philosophy that underpins them (brotherhood), could be construed as some of the elements of community wellbeing. Government obligations in this model are supportive of individual, family and community wellbeing. These obligations assume the form of transfer payments, facilitating economic growth and measures for equal opportunities, which could also be construed as contributing towards societal wellbeing.

At societal and national level, there have been attempts to redefine the HDI to construct an Islamic Human Development Index (IHDI). Similarly, there is the proposed Index of

Wellbeing for Muslim Countries. Both these latter, societal level constructs attempt to operationalise and measure indices that reflect Islamic values.

My definitional framework was developed within the context of Western secular society and the question was raised about the relevance of this model to other cultures (La Placa *et al.*, 2013a). I would hypothesise that within the context of a Muslim society, or any sub-group bound collectively by a distinct religious and world view, the wellbeing definitional framework, in such circumstances, would not be linear but multidimensional. It would also be characterised by a greater overlap between the circles representing the four domains of wellbeing. A complete convergence of the identified domains of wellbeing is not possible in practice, but it could be postulated that the ideological and policy goal would be to obtain as close a convergence as possible.

Understanding the wellbeing of Muslims is not possible without an account of the overarching nature of Islam. However, there is also substantial diversity between Muslim communities and countries, which defies the common stereotypes often pervasive in Western societies (Offenhauer, 2005). Better understanding of Islam, and Muslim communities, means going beyond religion and taking into account measures of human development, the geographic spread of Muslims, their distribution in different nation states with differing political/governance structures, ethnic and religious compositions, their experience of colonialism, natural resources endowment, and the extent of their integration into the global economy.

RESEARCH POINTER 10.1

- Compile a list of factors associated with religion that might be incorporated into a concept of wellbeing.

- How far should religious values and practices be incorporated into wellbeing?

FURTHER READING

Hamdi, T. I. and Al-Jadiry, A. M. H. (1979) *The Holy Qu'ran and the Psyche*. Paper given at the 12th Annual Convention of the Islamic Medical Association. Dallas, Texas.

Moghnie, L. and Kazarian, S.S. (2012) Subjective Happiness of Lebanese College Youth in Lebanon: Factorial Structure and Invariance of the Arabic Subjective Happiness Scale. *Social Indicators Research*, 109(2), 203–210.

The Holy Quran (2004) Arabic text, with English translation by Maulawi Sher Ali. Surrey, UK: Islamic International Publications.

11

CONCLUSION

Vincent La Placa, Anneyce Knight
and Allan McNaught

THEORISING WELLBEING

Wellbeing has emerged as a discursive late modern phenomenon, the uniqueness of which lies in the development of late modern capitalism. This process enables it to be articulated and used in modern policy discourse, and within less traditional contexts. As La Placa and Knight (2014) have argued, this historical process has witnessed wellbeing 'breaking' in to UK public health policy discourse as a discrete idea in its own right. As modern capitalism, consumerism and new forms of knowledge and relationships advance, individuals, national and global policy communities are less reliant on traditional patterns of relations and identities (Giddens, 1990; 1991). They have more choice to develop and revise previous actions and modes of thought. New means of devising individual and public/social policy requirements can be developed outside of tradition-bound contexts.

In fact, wellbeing has emerged as a key concept with which to understand and develop policies and strategies of change (as we mention initially in *Chapter 1*), in what Jameson (1984) also refers to as late-multinational capitalism. Under forms of early capitalism, culture and social institutions are driven through the economic medium, in the materialist object form of, for instance, machines, tools and production methods. This centres the self, community and policy around narrow economic concepts and meanings, related to, for example, work, materialism and economism. Capacity to apply different meanings and relations is limited in early capitalism as a result. In late capitalism, however, relations and meanings are more changeable and diffused as enhanced knowledge enables us to change and disseminate different meanings and ways of developing the self and relating to others. This displaces meanings and unties them from traditional economic relations. Wellbeing has emerged not only as a result of the decline of traditional economic structures, but also because of the potential to create and disseminate it through, for example, new technologies, developments in leisure, the mass media, and new ways of constructing the self and its location in broader relations. New concepts of wellbeing are a critical response to change, which enable individuals to construct meanings and relations outside of traditional and material forms (although the economy remains a fundamental domain of wellbeing). Tradition-bound economic modes no longer solely reproduce cultural discourses and symbols. Rather, through increased use of technology and non-economic discourses, new ways of constructing cultures emerge and reproduce concepts of wellbeing.

The emergence of wellbeing and the debates generated throughout this book constitute an example of this process, that of constructing and reframing new means of defining, studying and applying wellbeing. Wellbeing represents a new and discursive response to social and economic change, producing and realigning relations and adapting to new situations and events in the late modern world, as identified in *Chapters 2* and *3*, which focus on epistemological and theoretical issues around wellbeing. In addition, debates within this book, whether they circulate around wellbeing and minority groups (*Chapter 6*), wellbeing and demographic change (*Chapter 7*) or wellbeing and the physical environment (*Chapter 9*), are representations of, but also responses to change, with which individuals and societies are confronted in their day-to-day lives.

Similarly, the concept of 'life politics' (Giddens, 1990; 1991) has emerged over the last three decades within the social and behavioural sciences. Before modernity, there was 'emancipatory politics', whereby individuals and groups strived to liberate themselves collectively from constraints and structures that adversely influenced and governed their lives. The suffragettes, trade unions, and the lesbian and gay movement are examples of this. Life politics, however, concerns us more with contemporary personal choice and lifestyle, and the processes from which we construct our lives and identities within a framework of personal responses and choices to suit lifestyles and wellbeing. By constructing 'inner authenticity' and a sense of grounded 'self' and 'wellbeing', individuals diminish the effects of constant change and flux, resulting from modernity and instability. As a result, the study and application of wellbeing are significant in life politics, as are the ways we choose to maximise wellbeing and potentially construct a sense of security.

The experience of individual wellbeing is tied up with the experience of modernity and its rupture of traditionally embedded modes of thought and behaviour. However, as we have seen throughout this book, wellbeing transcends the individual and should theoretically and epistemologically account for wider local and social determinants, for example, families and communities (*Chapter 8*). Individuals construct wellbeing through lifestyle politics, but this is often enhanced or constrained through a web of socio-cultural structures. Individuals reflexively construct wellbeing and self-actualisation (and indeed health), but the wider and historical processes that aid or hinder this can be separate and encourage new ways of defining and collectively enhancing wellbeing.

Bagguley (1999) argues that there is little distinction between life and emancipatory politics. For example, self-actualisation itself often entails the use of collective action to improve and enhance socio-economic conditions and therefore wellbeing. Community development, community action and enhanced participation of people within the wider public health structure, constitute examples of this. Therefore, wellbeing must be studied and applied on both subjective and objective levels to view it in its entirety and complexity, recognising that both individual agency and wider circumstances are produced in interaction with one another and afford individuals and groups opportunities and challenges in changing their own lives and in collective transformation. As *Chapter 5* demonstrates, issues around housing, health, wellbeing and social care are multi-dimensional and solutions incorporate various key discursive and structural elements that reinforce one another, generating multiple processes and strategies towards individual and collective wellbeing.

The social and economic determinants, cultural processes and psycho-social outcomes of wellbeing are particularly relevant to prevent it being solely politicised and therefore weakening its richness, complexity and potential. Walker and Longley (2012) contend that wellbeing has appeal across the political spectrum. For example, emphasis on life politics may appeal to those who have political affiliations with the right, particularly with the individualistic conceptions of self and identity; references, however, to citizenship rights and happiness, regardless of income and status, are often appealing to those on the left of the political spectrum. However, the concept of wellbeing (as a discursive and analytical construct) is not effectively utilised, for example, if defined singularly and appropriated solely with reference to political appeal. For example, such divisions may lead wellbeing to be perceived through a dualistic lens as either 'individual psychology' or 'collective struggles against economic inequalities', reducing it to the realm of either the 'psychological' or 'economic'. Not only is this reductionist, but it works against policy makers' and healthcare practitioners' ability to work out, for instance, how wellbeing might be constructed through individual self-actualisation which might be affected by collective processes, thought and actions.

Clearly, the foregoing chapters suggest alternative means of capturing wellbeing beyond dualistic categories. *Chapter 3*, for example, argues the potential need to view collective processes beyond traditional economism, to collectivities grounded within new forms of exchange, relationships and social changes in late modern capitalism. This unties wellbeing from methodological individualism, but also focuses on how group or collective wellbeing can be constructed through competition and differentiation from other groups and interests. It is not to automatically assume that individual and collective wellbeing will be enhanced through either greater economic equality or 'social engineering'. Neither does it suggest that pure self-interest and individual free will drive wellbeing and policies to enhance it. Through developing and experimenting with new ways of defining and applying concepts of wellbeing, we lessen the risk that it will be reduced to a singular and narrow category and increase the potential of a multiple context-bound application.

WELLBEING IN POLICY MAKING AND PRACTICE

The concept of wellbeing as a category to produce policy discourse and development has been criticised for various reasons (Walker and Longley, 2012). For instance, Layard (2009) questions the prioritising of happiness and wellbeing, compared with other potential indicators often perceived as 'good'. Jordan (2006) questions whether we can adequately know what wellbeing is and what is conducive to it, particularly in developed economies, where the values of consumer choice and personal responsibility prevail. Wellbeing will always be weakened or even stalled within economies that measure happiness and quality of life with reference solely to economic growth and increased consumerism (Jordan, 2010). The contested nature of wellbeing (La Placa *et al.*, 2013a) itself inevitably brings about challenges and disagreements as to where and how concepts of wellbeing and happiness are relevant to people in their day-to-day lives and how they should be applied in policy and practice.

A key theme arising from this book is the challenge to policy makers and healthcare professionals of designing policies and interventions that make wellbeing seem 'real' and 'relevant' to the population as a whole and provide adequate responses to the above criticisms. For example, *Chapter 10* has reflected upon religious meaning and its association with a definition and measurement of wellbeing, which is relevant to the groups and individuals in question. Wellbeing must be made to 'mean' and 'feel' something among lay people, and be perceived to be relevant to policy and public health outcomes, among professionals. Despite its limitations, biomedicine does at least contain the capacity to deliver outcomes that are perceived as real and relevant; for instance, in the palliation of pain and physical illness (regardless of whether it pays attention to wellbeing and other social and relational determinants). Wellbeing should be a two-way relationship between lay populations and professionals. It needs grounding in a 'double hermeneutics' (Giddens, 1993), understood by all communities, if it is not to be passed off as a 'fad' or abandoned by future governments. Concepts and ideas used by social scientists and policy makers can be employed by lay agents, capable of transforming their own communities and environments, as well as individual lives.

Jordan (2010) suggests that community and 'grassroots' activities and services (much like those described in *Chapters 8* and *9*), which place value on social interaction, relations, trust and solidarity between people, can significantly enhance wellbeing and form the basis of wider national policies. Business, government, voluntary and community organisations may benefit from increased economic efficiency and consumerism, but this is experienced more positively where 'cultures' of wellbeing are encouraged simultaneously. For example, social and community enterprise activities around sport and music can produce both economic and social value (Jordan, 2010). These can create cultural and economic resources which reach across individuals and community and enhance wellbeing. Experts, professionals and lay people can be involved, forming personal and professional bonds and developing means of strengthening individual ability to cope and learn, whilst simultaneously enhancing collective wellbeing. It is a form of 'productivism' based upon service, sustainability and investment in individuals' economic and social capital. Clearly, the creation of local Health and Wellbeing Boards (*Chapter 4*) can develop and embed community and grassroots activities, which involve both professional and lay individuals (La Placa and Knight, 2014).

Another challenge lies in policy makers' and healthcare practitioners' ability to generate discourses and interventions in an environment where traditional methods and means of viewing, for instance, 'wellbeing', 'satisfaction' and 'happiness' change, often dramatically; but also where current modes of Anglo-Saxon capitalism have remained largely unchanged, despite recent austerity and fluxes in modern economic systems. We recognise that wellbeing policies and interventions can and will be affected by the financial and structural conditions within the current economic climate.

However, Jordan (2010) argues that the current economic climate can and does open up opportunities for individuals and governments to develop policies based upon interdependence, pooling of resources, sharing of risks, and the need to encourage cooperation in strengthening solidarity and trust. An example of this is the increasing realisation that local cooperation and innovation in the development of health and wellbeing activities can strengthen ties and embed people in the social and economic life of the community. We believe these developments can enhance wellbeing as a useful and analytical category in informing policies and improving the lives of individuals and groups in the current economic climate. In fact, due to the contingency and complexity of wellbeing, the category may well be affected and developed by both economic and non-economic drivers, sometimes operating in tandem. Technology, globalisation, and the encouragement of local and community identities and services throughout the UK, will form important drivers, as will developments in the production of targeted and population-based wellbeing interventions, which incorporate and use these drivers. We also argue that concepts of wellbeing can actually be seen to drive economic and social policy (and not the other way around), for instance, in the policy makers' attempts to measure and formulate policy in regards to wellbeing (however it is defined).

These debates also present further challenges towards, for example, choices between local and generic wellbeing interventions and the relationships (economic and non-economic) between different and competing segments of the UK population. The globalisation of culture and economies may also witness a shift to global definitions of wellbeing, adding another complex, but rich discourse to the policy making process and establishing wellbeing as a core concept in the 21st century. Jordan (2006) argues that "global cosmopolitanism", and a shared sense of international cooperation, afford more opportunities for social justice and development than sole reliance on national policies. Indeed as Chirico (2013) posits, globalisation is as much part of the subjective sense of self as it is economic and technological. For example, it enables the possibility that one feels a sense of belonging with universal humanity beyond that of the individual. It is by developing wellbeing as an analytical and conceptual category, fit for application, which can assist policy makers and healthcare practitioners to decide the effects of such strategies, particularly their relevance to context and defined need. We hope this book helps in that process.

REFERENCES

Abdel-Khalek, A. M. (2004) Happiness Among Kuwaiti College Students. *Journal of Happiness Studies*, 5: 93–97.

Abdel-Khalek, A. M. (2006a) Happiness, Health, and Religiosity: Significant Relations. *Mental Health, Religion and Culture*, 9(1): 85–97.

Abdel-Khalek, A. M. (2006b) Measuring Happiness with a Single Item Scale. *Social Behavior and Personality*, 34: 139–150.

Abdel-Khalek, A. M. (2008) Religiosity, Health and Wellbeing Among Kuwaiti Personnel. *Psychological Reports*, 102: 181–184.

Abdel-Khalek, A. M. (2010) Quality of Life, Subjective Wellbeing, and Religiosity in Muslim College Students. *Quality of Life Research*, 19, 1133–1143.

Abdelhak, S. and Sulaiman, J. (2001) *The Importance of Islamic Values in the Enhancement of Household's Wellbeing: A Study of Poverty Alleviation in the Malaysian State of Pulau Pinang*, Eighth International Conference on Islamic Economics and Finance, Doha: Qatar.

Ackoff, R. (1974) *Redesigning the Future: A Systems Approach to Societal Problems*. New York: Wiley.

Aflakseir, A. (2012) Religiosity, Personal Meaning and Psychological Wellbeing: A Study Among Muslim Students in England. *Pakistan Journal of Social and Clinical Psychology*, 9(2), 27–31.

Ahmad, K. (1959) *Towards Understanding Islam*. Available at: **www.sa.niu.edu/msa/books/ towardsunderstandingislam.pdf** [accessed 5 December 2013].

Aked, J., Mark, N., Cordon, C. and Thompson, S. (2008) *Five Ways to Wellbeing Report*. London: The New Economics Foundation Centre for Wellbeing.

Al-Ghazzali, I. (1910/2005) *The Alchemy of Happiness*. New York: Cosimo.

Alderson, P. (1998) The Importance of Theories in Health Care. *British Medical Journal*, 317 (7164), 1007–1010.

Alexander, J. C. (2004) Towards a Theory of Cultural Trauma. In: Alexander, J. C., Eyerman, R., Giesen, B., Smelser, N. J. and Sztompka, P. (Eds) *Cultural Trauma and Collective Identity*. Berkeley, CA: University of California Press.

Allen, J. (2008) *Older People and Wellbeing*. London: Institute for Public Policy Research.

Andrews, J. and Molyneux, P. (Aus) with Swan, A. and Bell, P. (Eds) (2013) *Dementia: Finding Housing Solutions*. London: National Housing Federation. Online. Available at: **www.housing.org.uk/publications/browse/dementia-finding-housing-solutions** [accessed 11 December 2013].

Ashbullby, K. and White, M. (2012) *Being Beside the Seaside is Good for your Emotional Wellbeing*. Online. Available at: **www.ecehh.org/news/being-beside-seaside-good-your-emotional-wellbeing** [accessed 20 May 2013].

Asthana, S. and Halliday, J. (2006) *What Works in Tackling Health Inequalities? Pathways, Policies and Practice Through the Lifecourse*. Bristol: Policy Press.

Bagguley, P. (1999) Beyond Emancipation? The Reflexivity of Social Movements. In: O'Brien, M., Penna, S. and Hay, C. (Eds) *Theorising Modernity: Reflexivity, Environment and Identity in Giddens' Social Theory*. London: Longman.

Bancroft, A. (2005) *Roma and Gypsy – Travellers in Europe: Modernity, Race, Space and Exclusion*. Gateshead: Athenaeum Press.

Barratt, C., Green, G., Speed, E. and Price, P. (2012a) *Understanding the Relationship between Mental Health and Bedsits in a Seaside Town*. Essex: Tendring District Council and University of Essex.

Barratt, C., Kitcher, C. and Stewart, J. (2012b) Beyond Safety to Wellbeing: How Local Authorities Can Mitigate the Mental Health Risks of Living Houses in Multiple Occupation, *Journal of Environmental Health Research*, 12(1), 39–50.

Bartley, M. (2004) *Health Inequality: An Introduction to Theories, Concepts and Methods*. Cambridge: Polity Press.

Batchelor, D. A. F. (2006) A New Islamic Rating Index of Well-being for Muslim Countries. *Islam and Civilizational Renewal*, 4(2), 188–214.

Beck, U. (1992) *Risk Society: Towards a New Modernity*. London: Sage.

Behan, D. (2011) Letter (dated 20 June 2011) from Director General for Social Care, Local Government and Care Partnerships to All Leaders and Chief Executives of Local Authorities.

Belton, B. (2005) *Gypsy and Traveller Ethnicity: The Social Generation of an Ethnic Phenomenon.* London: Routledge.

Benzeval, M., Judge, K. and Whitehead, M. (1995). *Tackling Inequalities in Health: An Agenda for Action.* London: King's Fund.

Bingham, J. (2013) Schools told to run parenting classes and measure happiness. *The Daily Telegraph.* Online. Available at: **www.telegraph.co.uk/education/educationnews/ 10331729/Schools-told-to-run-parenting-classes-and-measure-happiness.html** [accessed 1 October 2013].

Binley, A., Cheshire, S. and Bridgwood, A. (2008) *Green Spaces and Sustainable Communities (GSSC) and Transforming Waste Evaluation Summary.* Northampton: Belmont Press.

Bochel, C. (2009) Exploring the Boundaries of Social Policy. In: Bochel, H., Bochel, C., Page, R. and Sykes, R. (Eds) *Social Policy: Themes, Issues and Debates* (2nd edn). Harlow: Pearson Education Limited.

Bok, S. (2010) *Exploring Happiness: From Aristotle to Brain Science.* New Haven, CT: Yale University Press.

Bourne, P. A. (2010) A Conceptual Framework of Wellbeing in Some Western Nations (A Review Article): Current Research. *Journal of Social Sciences,* 2(1), 15–23.

Calkin, S. and Ford, S. (2011) Beefed up Health and Wellbeing Boards Extend Council Powers. *Health Services Journal.* Online. Available at: **www.hsj.co.uk/news/policy/councils-gain-power-via-beefed-up-health-and-wellbeing-boards/5031167.article** [accessed 2 April 2014].

Cameron, E., Mathers, J. and Parry, J. (2006) Health and Well-being: Questioning the Use of Health Concepts in Public Health Policy and Practice. *Critical Public Health,* 16(4), 347–354.

Caras, C. (2003) *Religiosity/Spirituality and Subjective Wellbeing.* B. App. Sci. (Hon) Thesis. Melbourne: Deakin University.

Care and Repair England (2012) *Making your Home a Better Place to Live with Dementia.* Online. Available at: **www.careandrepair-england.org.uk/homefromhospital/pdf/live_ with_dementia.pdf** [accessed 26 June 2013].

Care Quality Commission (2011) *Dignity and Nutrition for Older People: 2011 Inspection Programme.* Online. Available at: **www.cqc.org.uk/public/reports-surveys-and-reviews/themed-inspections/dignity-and-nutrition-older-people/dignity-a-1** [accessed 31 May 2013].

Care Quality Commission (2013a) *Time to Listen In NHS Hospitals: Dignity and Nutrition Inspection Programme 2012.* Online. Available at: **www.cqc.org.uk/sites/default/files/media/ documents/time_to_listen_-_nhs_hospitals_main_report_tag.pdf** [accessed 31 May 2013].

Care Quality Commission (2013b) *Time to Listen in Care Homes: Dignity and Nutrition Inspection Programme 2012*. Online. Available at: **www.cqc.org.uk/sites/default/files/media/documents/time_to_listen_-_care_homes_main_report_tag.pdf** [accessed 31 May 2013].

Cemlyn, S., Greenfields, M., Burnett, S., Matthews, Z. and Whitwell, C. (2009) *Inequalities Experienced by Gypsy and Traveller Communities: A Review*. London: Equality and Human Rights Commission.

Chanan, C. and Miller, C. (2013) *Rethinking Community Practice: Developing Transformative Neighbourhoods*. Bristol: Policy Press.

Checkland, P. and Poulter, J. (2006) *Learning for Action: A Short Definitive Account of Soft Systems Methodology and its Use for Practitioners, Teachers and Students*. Chichester: Wiley.

Checkland, P. and Scholes, J. (1990) *Soft Systems Methodology in Action*. Chichester: Wiley.

Chirico, J. (2013) *Globalization: Prospects and Problems*. London: Sage.

Clatworthy, J. (2012) *Gardening and Wellbeing*. Doctoral dissertation, Canterbury Christ Church University, Kent (unpublished).

Coburn, D. (2004) Beyond the Income Inequality Hypothesis: Class, Neo-liberalism, and Health Inequalities. *Social Science and Medicine*, 58, 41–56.

Community Care (2008) *Personalisation*. Online. Available at: **www.communitycare.co.uk/2008/08/07/personalisation/** [accessed 1 December 2013].

Comte, A. (1975) Plan of the Scientific Operations Necessary for Reorganizing Society. In: G. Lenzer (Ed.). *Auguste Comte and Positivism: The Essential Writings*. New York: Harper Torchbooks.

Cowie, J. and Mages, L. (2011) Communities and Health: A Scottish Health Perspective. In: Porter, E. and Coles, L. (Eds) *Policy and Strategy for Improving Health and Wellbeing*. Exeter: Learning Matters.

Crew, D. (2007) *The Tenant's Dilemma*. Crosby: Formby and District Citizens Advice Bureau.

Cummins, R. A., Eckersley, R., Pallant, J., Van Vugt, J. and Misajohn, R. (2003) The Australian Unity Wellbeing Index. *Social Indicators Research*, 64, 159–190.

Dalmayr, F. R. (1986) Democracy and Post-Modernism. *Human Studies*, 10(1), 143–170.

Davey Smith, G. (2003) *Health Inequalities: Lifecourse Approaches*. Bristol: Policy Press.

Dawes, S., Cresswell, A. and Pardo, T. (2009) From "Need to Know" to "Need to Share": Tangled Problems, Information Boundaries, and the Building of Public Sector Knowledge Networks. *Public Administration Review*, 69(3), 392–402.

Department for Environment, Food and Rural Affairs (DEFRA) (2009) *Sustainable Development Indicators in your Pocket.* London: DEFRA.

Department for Environment, Transport and the Regions (DETR) (2000) *Urban White Paper: Our Towns and Cities: The Future – Delivering an Urban Renaissance.* London: HMSO.

Department of Health (2001) *National Service Framework for Older People.* Online. Available at: **www.gov.uk/government/publications/quality-standards-for-care-services-for-older-people** [accessed 31 May 2013].

Department of Health (2009) *New Horizons: A Shared Vision for Mental Health.* London: Department of Health.

Department of Health (2010a) *Our Health and Wellbeing.* London: Department of Health.

Department of Health (2010b) *Healthy Lives, Healthy People: Our Strategy for Public Health in England.* London: Department of Health.

Department of Health (2011) *Early Implementers of Health and Wellbeing Boards Announced.* Online. Available at **http://healthandcare.dh.gov.uk/early-implementers-of-health-and-wellbeing-boards-announced/** [accessed 5 July 2011].

Department of Health (2012a) *Local Healthwatch: A Strong Voice for People – The Policy Explained.* London: Department of Health.

Department of Health (2012b) *A Summary Table of the Duties and Powers Introduced by the Health and Social Care Act 2012 Relevant to JSNAs and JHWSs.* Online. Available at: **www.wp.dh.gov.uk/publications/files/2012/07/Table-of-duties-and-powers.pdf** [accessed 5 July 2013].

Department of Health and NHS Commissioning Board (2012) *Compassion in Practice, Nursing, Midwifery and Care Staff: Our Vision and Strategy.* London: The Stationery Office.

Depledge, M. and Bird, W. (2009) The Blue Gym: Health and Wellbeing from our Coasts. *Marine Pollution Bulletin,* 58, 947–948.

Dharamsi, S., Espinoza, N., Cramer, C., Amin, M., Bainbridge, L. and Poole, G. (2010) Nurturing Social Responsibility. *Medical Teacher,* 32, 905–911.

Dhesi, S. (2014) *Exploring how Health and Wellbeing Boards are Tackling Health Inequalities, With a Focus on the Role of Environmental Health.* PhD thesis, University of Manchester, in press.

Diener, E. (2009a) *The Science of Well-Being: The Collected Works of Ed Diener.* New York: Springer Dordrecht.

Diener, E. (2009b) *Culture and Well-Being: The Collected Works of Ed Diener.* New York: Springer Dordrecht.

Diener, E. and Diener, M. (1995) Cross-Cultural Correlates of Life Satisfaction and Self-Esteem. *Journal of Personality and Social Psychology,* 68(4), 653–663.

Diener, E., Diener, M. and Diener, C. (1995) Factors Predicting the Subjective Well-being of Nations. *Journal of Personality and Social Psychology,* 69(5), 851–864.

Diener, E. and Seligman, M. E. (2002) Very Happy People. *Psychology Science,* 13(1), 81–84.

Diener, E., Oishi, S. and Lucas, R. E. (2003) Personality, Culture, and Subjective Well-being: Emotional and Cognitive Evaluations of Life. *Annual Review of Psychology,* 54, 403.

Dooris, M. (2004) Joining Up Settings for Health: A Valuable Investment for Strategic Partnerships. *Critical Public Health,* 14(1), 49–61.

Emanuel, S. (1993) Meeting the Needs of HMO Tenants. *Environmental Health,* January 1993, 5–7.

English Heritage and Urban Practitioners (2007) An Asset and a Challenge: Heritage and Regeneration in Coastal Towns in England: Final report. Online. Available at: **www.helm.org.uk/guidance-library/asset-challenge-heritage-regeneration-coastal-towns-england/Coastal-Towns-Report3.pdf** [accessed 17 July 2013].

Europa (2013) *About the year: 2012 – European Year for Active Ageing and Solidarity Between Generations.* Online. Available at: **http://europa.eu/ey2012/ey2012main.jsp?catId=971&langId=en** [accessed 26 May 2013].

European Commission (2008) *European Pact for Mental Health and Well-being.* Online. Available at: **http://ec.europa.eu/health/mental_health/policy/statements/index_en.htm** [accessed 29 May 2013].

European Commission (2013) *Ageing policy.* Online. Available at: **http://ec.europa.eu/health/ageing/policy/index_en.htm** [accessed 26 May 2013].

Evans, D. and Killoran, A. (2000) Tackling Health Inequalities Through Partnership Working: Learning from a Realistic Evaluation. *Critical Public Health,* 10(2), 125–140.

Ferguson, I., Lavalette, M. and Mooney, G. (2002) *Rethinking Welfare: A Critical Perspective.* London: Sage.

Fitzpatrick, M. M. (2011) Health and Wellbeing Boards. *British Journal of General Practice,* 61(587), 406.

Foresight Mental Capital and Wellbeing Project (2008) *Final Project Report – Executive Summary.* London: The Government Office for Science.

Forestry Commission (2013) THERAPI project. Online. Available at: **www.forestry.gov.uk/pdf/Ion-casestudiesitherapi/$FILE/Ion-casestudies-therapi-pdf** [accessed 30 September 2013].

Francis, R. (2013) *Final Report of the Independent Inquiry into the Care Provided by Mid Staffordshire NHS Foundation Trust*. Online. Available at: **www.midstaffsinquiry.com/pressrelease.html** [accessed 8 July 2013].

Fredrickson, B. L. (2002) How Does Religion Benefit Health and Well-being?: Are Positive Emotions Active Ingredients? *Psychological Inquiry*, 13(3), 209–212.

Fulton, R. (2010) *Better Health Briefing* (21): *Ethnic Monitoring: Is Health Equality Possible Without It?* London: Race Equality Foundation.

Giddens, A. (1990) *The Consequences of Modernity*. Cambridge: Polity Press.

Giddens, A. (1991) *Modernity and Self-identity: Self and Society in the Late Modern Age*. Cambridge: Polity Press.

Giddens, A. (1993) *New Rules of Sociological Method* (2nd edn). Cambridge: Polity Press.

Gidley, B. and Rooke, A. (2008) *Learning from the Local: The Newtown Neighbourhood Project: Final Report*. London: Goldsmiths College, University of London.

Gilbert, P. (2013) *The Compassionate Mind*. London: Constable and Robinson.

Glasby, J., Dickinson, H. and Smith, J. (2010) Creating NHS Local: The Relationship Between English Local Government and the National Health Service. *Social Policy and Administration*, 44(3), 244–264.

Glendinning, C. (2002) Partnerships Between Health and Social Services: Developing a Framework for Evaluation. *Policy and Politics*, 30(1), 115–127.

Goward, P., Repper, J., Appleton, L. and Hagan, T. (2006) Crossing Boundaries: Identifying and Meeting the Mental Health Needs of Gypsies and Travellers. *Journal of Mental Health*, 15(3), 315–327.

Graham, C. (2011) *The Pursuit of Happiness: An Economy of Well-Being*. Washington DC: The Brookings Institution Press.

Graham, H. (2009) Health Inequalities, Social Determinants and Public Health Policy. *Policy and Politics*, 37, 463–479.

Greenfields, M. and Smith, D. (2010) Housed Gypsy/Travellers, Social Segregation and the Reconstruction of Communities. *Housing Studies*, 28(3), 397–412.

Griffin, J. (2002) *Well-Being: Its Meaning, Measurement and Moral Importance*. Oxford: Oxford University Press.

Habermas, J. (1990) *The Philosophical Discourse of Modernity: Twelve Lectures*. Cambridge: Policy Press.

Habermas, J. (1992) *The Structural Transformation of the Public Sphere: An Inquiry into a Category of Bourgeois Society*. Cambridge: Policy Press.

Habgood, V. (2011) Environment and Wellbeing. In: Knight, A. and McNaught, A. (Eds) *Understanding Wellbeing: An Introduction for Students and Practitioners of Health and Social Care*. Banbury: Lantern Publishing.

Hamdi, T. I. and Al-Jadiry, A. M. H. (1979) *The Holy Qu'ran and the Psyche*. Paper given at the 12th Annual Convention of the Islamic Medical Association, Dallas, Texas.

Hammond, C. (2004) Impacts of Lifelong Learning Upon Emotional Resilience, Psychological and Mental Health: Fieldwork Evidence. *Oxford Review of Education*, 30, 551–568.

Haponava, T. and Al-Jibouri, S. (2012) Proposed System for Measuring Project Performance Using Processed-Based Key Performance Indicators. *Journal of Management in Engineering*, DOI: 10.1061/(ASCE)ME.1943-5479.0000078.

Harding, E. and Kane, M. (2011) Joint Strategic Needs Assessment: Reconciling New Expectations with Reality. *Journal of Integrated Care*, 19(6), 37–44.

Heifetz, R. and Laurie, D. (1997) The Work of Leadership. *Harvard Business Review*, 75(1), 124–134.

Helliwell, J., Layard, R. and Sachs, J. (2012) *World Happiness Report*. New York: Earth Institute, Columbia University.

Helliwell, J., Layard, R. and Sachs, J. (2013) *World Happiness Report*. New York: Earth Institute, Columbia University.

Hendrie Anto, M. B. (2009) Introducing an Islamic Human Development Index (I-HDI) to Measure Development in OIC Countries. *Islamic Economic Studies*, 19(2), 69–95.

Hill, M. and Honey, A. (2010) *Report to Communities Policy Overview and Scrutiny Committee*. Thanet Council. Online. Available at: **http://democracy.kent.gov.uk/documents/s14311/item%20B7%20-%20Margate%20Task%20Force.pdf** [accessed 17 December 2011].

Hills, J. and Stewart, K. (2005) *A More Equal Society? New Labour, Poverty, Inequality and Exclusion*. Bristol: Policy Press.

HM Government (1999) *Health Act 1999*. London: The Stationery Office.

HM Government (2013) Care Bill. Online. Available at: **www.official-documents.gov.uk/document/cm86/8627/8627.asp** [accessed 26 May 2013].

Hollander, J. A. and Einwohner, R. L. (2004) Conceptualizing Resistance. *Sociological Forum*, 19(4), 533–554.

Hopkins, R. J. (2011) Food Poverty: Living in Hotels and Guesthouses Without Access to Adequate Kitchen Facilities. *Journal of Environmental Health Research*, 11(2), 67–96.

Horkheimer, M. and Adorno, T. W. (1972) *Dialectic of Enlightenment*. New York: Herder and Herder.

House of Commons Communities and Local Government Committee (2007) *Coastal Towns: Second Report of Session 2006–07*. London: The Stationery Office.

Humphries, R., Galea, A., Sonola, L. and Mundle, C. (2012) *Health and Wellbeing Boards: System Leaders or Talking Shops?* London: The Kings Fund.

Hunt, J. (2013) *Speech: Primary Care and the Modern Family Doctor*. Online. Available at: **www.gov.uk/government/speeches/primary-care-and-the-modern-family-doctor** [accessed 2 June 2013].

Hunter, D. (2009) Leading for Health and Wellbeing: The Need for a New Paradigm. *Journal of Public Health*, 31(2), 202–204.

Hunter, D. J., Marks, L. and Smith, K. E. (2010) *The Public Health System in England*. Bristol: Policy Press.

Jameson, F. (1984) *The Postmodern Condition*. Minneapolis: University of Minnesota University.

John, M. (2012) Wellbeing and Older People. In: Walker, P. and John, M. (Eds) *From Public Health to Wellbeing: The New Drive for Policy and Action*. Basingstoke: Palgrave.

Johns, R. (2011) From State Welfare to a Mixed Economy: The Era of Community Care. In: Johns, R. (Ed.). *Social Work, Social Policy and Older People*. Exeter: Learning Matters.

Jones, O. (2011) *Chavs: The Demonisation of the Working Class*. London: Verso.

Jones–Devitt, S and Smith, L. (2007) *Critical Thinking in Health and Social Care*. London: Sage.

Jordan, B. (2006) *Social Policy for the Twenty-First Century: New Perspectives, Big Issues*. Cambridge: Polity.

Jordan, B. (2008) *Welfare and Well-being: Social Value in Public Policy*. Bristol: Policy Press.

Jordan, B. (2010) *What's Wrong with Social Policy and How to Fix it*. Cambridge: Polity.

Kaldor, P., Hughes, P., Castle, K. and Bellamy, J. (2004) *Spirituality and Wellbeing in Australia*, NCLS Occasional Paper 6. Sydney: NCLS Research.

Kavanagh, D. (1990) *Thatcherism and British Politics: The End of Consensus*, (2nd edn). Oxford: Oxford University Press.

Kayani, N. (2009) Food, Health and Wellbeing. In: Stewart, J. and Cornish, Y. (Eds) *Professional Practice in Public Health*. Exeter: Reflect Press.

Kemp, P. A. (2011) Low-Income Tenants in the Private Rental Housing Market. *Housing Studies*, 26(7–8), 1019–1034.

Kemp, P. A. and Keoghan, M. (2001) Movement Into and Out of the Private Rented Sector in England. *Housing Studies*, 16(1), 21–37.

Kent County Council (2011a) *Here's History: Kent Margate*. Online. Available at: **www. hereshistorykent.org.uk/DisplayArticle.cfm?placeID=290&categoryID=1&placename= Margate** [accessed 30 November 2011].

Kent County Council (2011b) *The Indices of Deprivation: Detailed Findings for Kent*. Kent: Kent County Council.

Kirkwood, T., Bond, J., May, C., McKeith, I. and Teh, M. (2008) *Mental Capital Through Life Challenge Report*. London: The Government Office for Science.

Knight, A. (2009) Meeting the Challenges of Poverty, Inequality and Social Exclusion. In: Stewart, J. and Cornish, Y. (Eds) *Professional Practice in Public Health*. Exeter: Reflect Press.

Knight, A. and Khan, Q. (2011) Spirituality and Wellbeing. In: Knight, A. and McNaught, A. (Eds) *Understanding Wellbeing: An Introduction for Students and Practitioners of Health and Social Care*. Banbury: Lantern Publishing.

Knight, A. and La Placa, V. (2013) Healthy Universities: Taking the University of Greenwich Healthy Universities Initiative Forward. *International Journal of Health Promotion and Education*, 51(1), 41–49.

Knight, A. and McNaught, A. (2011) Conclusion. In: Knight, A. and McNaught, A. (Eds) *Understanding Wellbeing: An Introduction for Students and Practitioners of Health and Social Care*. Banbury: Lantern Publishing.

Knight, A. and Stewart, J. (2013) Long Term Care of the Elderly: A Policy Perspective (UK). In: Mackova, M. (Ed.). *Long Term Care of the Elderly*. Pardubice, Czech Republic: University of Pardubice.

Kydd, A. (2009) Values: What Older People Told Us. In: Kydd, A., Duffy, T. and Duffy, R. (Eds) *The Care and Wellbeing of Older People*. Exeter: Reflect Press.

Kydd, A., Duffy, T. and Duffy, R. (Eds) (2009) *The Care and Wellbeing of Older People*. Exeter: Reflect Press.

Laird, L. D., Amer, M. M., Barnett, E. D. and Barnes, L. L. (2007) Muslim Patients and Health Disparities in the UK and the US. *Archive of Diseases in Childhood*, 92(10), 922–926.

La Placa, V. and Corlyon, J. (2013) Social Tourism and Organised Capitalism: Research, Policy and Practice. *Journal of Policy Research in Tourism, Leisure and Events,* 6(1), 66–79.

La Placa, V., McNaught, A. and Knight, A. (2013a) Discourse on Wellbeing in Research and Practice. *International Journal of Wellbeing,* 3(1), 116–125.

La Placa, V., McVey, D., MacGregor, E., Smith, A. and Scott, M. (2013b) The Contribution of Qualitative Research to the Healthy Foundations Life-stage Segmentation. *Critical Public Health,* DOI: 10.1080/09581596.2013.797068.

La Placa, V. and Knight, A. (2014) Wellbeing: Its Influence and Local Impact on Public Health, *Public Health,* 128(1), 38–42.

Larkin, M. (2013) *Health and Well-being Across the Life Course.* London: Sage.

Laungani, P. (2002) Stress, Trauma and Coping Strategies: Cross-Cultural Variations. *International Journal of Group Tensions,* 31(2), 127–154.

Layard, R. (2009) Afterword. In: Griffiths, S. and Reeves, R. (Eds) *Wellbeing: How to Lead the Good Life and What Government Should do to Help.* London: Social Market Foundation.

Lee, B. Y. and Newberg, A. B. (2005) Religion and Health: A Review and Critical Analysis. *Zygon,* 40(2), 443–468.

Lee, M. (2006) *Promoting Mental Health and Wellbeing in Later Life: A First Report from the UK Inquiry into Mental Health and Wellbeing in Later Life.* London: Mental Health Foundation and Age Concern.

Letwin, R. S. (1992) *An Anatomy of Thatcherism.* London: Fontana.

Lewis, C. A. (2002) Church Attendance and Happiness among Northern Irish Undergraduate Students: No Association. *Pastoral Psychology,* 50, 191–195.

Lewis, C. A., Lanigan, C., Joseph, S., and deFockert, J. (1997) Religiosity and Happiness: No Evidence for an Association Among Undergraduates. *Personality and Individual Differences,* 12, 119–121.

Llewellyn, A. (2009) Sociology and Ageing. In: Kydd, A., Duffy, T. and Duffy, R. (Eds) *The Care and Wellbeing of Older People.* Exeter: Reflect Press.

Lyotard, F. R. (1984) *The Postmodern Condition: A Report on Knowledge (Theory and History of Literature).* Manchester: Manchester University Press.

Maas, J., Verheij, R. A., Groenewegen, P. P., de Vries, S. and Spreeuwenberg, P. (2006) Green Space, Urbanity and Health: How Strong is the Relation? *Journal of Epidemiological Community Health,* 60, 587–592.

Mackenbach, J. P. (2010) Has the English Strategy to Reduce Health Inequalities Failed?

Social Science and Medicine, 71, 1249–1253.

Madrigal, C. R. (2008) *Acculturation, Ethnic Identity, Resilience, Self Esteem and General Wellbeing: A Psychosocial Study of Colombians in the United States.* Ann Arbor, MI: ProQuest LLC.

Margate Renewal Partnership (2009) *Dreamland Margate Sea Change Application: Proposal Support Document Equality Impact Assessment.* Margate: Margate Renewal Partnership.

Marmot, M. and Wilkinson, R. (2006) *Social Determinants of Health* (2nd edn). Oxford: Oxford University Press.

Marmot, M. G., Allen, J., Goldblatt, P., Boyce, T., McNeish, D., Grady, M. and Geddes, I. (2010) *Fair Society, Healthy Lives: Strategic Review of Health Inequalities in England Post-2010.* London: University College London.

Masir, G. A. and Adam, N. J. (1995) *The Way to Happiness.* Al-Batha: Cooperative Office for Call and Guidance.

Mathews, G. and Izquierdo, C. (2009) *Pursuits of Happiness: Well-Being in Anthropological Perspective.* New York: Berghahn Books.

Mayall, D. (2004) *Gypsy Identities 1500–2000: From Egyptians and Moon-men to the Ethnic Romany.* London: Routledge.

McKevitt, C and Wolfe, C. (2002) What Does Quality of Life Mean? The Views of Health Care Professionals. *Quality in Ageing,* 3(1), 12–19.

McKevitt, C., Redfern, J., La Placa, V. and Wolfe, C. D. A. (2003) Defining and Using Quality of Life: A Survey of Health Care Professionals. *Clinical Rehabilitation,* 17, 865–870.

McNaught, A. (2011) Defining Wellbeing. In: Knight, A. and McNaught, A. (Eds) *Understanding Wellbeing: An Introduction for Students and Practitioners of Health and Social Care.* Banbury: Lantern Publishing.

McVeigh, R. (1997) Theorising Sedentarism: The Roots of Anti-nomadism. In: Acton, T. (Ed.). *Gypsy Politics and Traveller Identity.* Hertford: University of Hertford Press.

Mehmet, N. (2011) Ethics and Wellbeing. In: Knight, A. and McNaught, A. (Eds) *Understanding Wellbeing: An Introduction for Students and Practitioners of Health and Social Care.* Banbury: Lantern Publishing.

Mihr, I. A. (1990) *Islam Happiness Sufism.* Bloomington: iUniverse.

Mitchell, R., Shaw, M. and Dorling, D. (2000) *Inequalities in Life and Death. What if Britain were More Equal?* Bristol: Policy Press.

Moghnie, L. and Kazarian, S. S. (2012) Subjective Happiness of Lebanese College Youth in Lebanon: Factorial Structure and Invariance of the Arabic Subjective Happiness Scale. *Social Indicators Research,* 109(2), 203–210.

Monk, A., and Howard, S. (1998) Methods and Tools: The Rich Picture: A Tool for Reasoning about Work Context. *Interactions,* 5(2), 21–30.

Moreno-Leguizamon, C. and Spigner, C. (2009) Theory, Research and Practice in Public Health. In: Stewart, J. and Cornish, Y. (Eds) *Professional Practice in Public Health.* Exeter: Reflect Press.

Moreno-Leguizamon, C. and Spigner, C. (2011) Monitoring and Evaluating Wellbeing Projects. In: Knight, A. and McNaught, A. (Eds) *Understanding Wellbeing: An Introduction for Students and Practitioners of Health and Social Care.* Banbury: Lantern Publishing.

Moosavi, S. M. (2005) Looking for Happiness: Happiness According to Psychology and Islam (part 1). *Hoda Magazine,* 1(1), 31–33.

Moosavi, S. M. (2006a) Looking for Happiness: Psychology and Happiness (part 2). *Hoda Magazine,* 1(2), 1–4.

Moosavi, S. M. (2006b) Looking for Happiness: Happiness According to Psychology and Islam (part 3). *Hoda Magazine,* 1(3), 3–6.

Moosavi, S. M. (2008) Happiness According to Psychology and Islam: The Ingredients of Happiness (part 4). *Hoda Magazine,* 1(4), 2–5.

Morrow, V. (2001) *Networks and Neighbourhoods: Children's and Young People's Perspectives.* London: Health Development Agency.

Murty, S., Franzini, L., Low, M. D. and Swint, J. M. (2009) Policies/Programs for Reducing Health Inequalities by Tackling Nonmedical Determinants of Health in the United Kingdom. *Social Science Quarterly,* 90(5), 1403–1422.

National Allotment Society (2013) *Brief History of Allotments.* Online. Available at: **www.nsalg.org.uk/allotment-info/brief-history-of-allotments/** [accessed 30 September 2013].

National Institute for Health and Clinical Excellence (2006) *Dementia QS1.* Online. Available at: **http://guidance.nice.org.uk/QS1** [accessed 31 May 2013].

Netto, G. (2008) Vulnerability to Homelessness, Use of Services and Homelessness Prevention in Black and Minority Ethnic Communities. *Housing Studies,* 21(4), 581–601.

New Economics Foundation (2008) *The Five Ways to Wellbeing.* Online. Available at: **www.neweconomics.org/projects/entry/five-ways-to-well-being** [accessed 30 September 2013].

NHS (2012) *Tai Chi and Heart Health in Older People.* Online. Available at: **www.nhs.uk/news/2012/04april/Pages/tai-chi-chuan-and-heath-health-old-people.aspx** [accessed 13 October 2013].

NHS England (2013) *Action Area 1: Helping People to Stay Independent, Maximising Well-being and Improving Health Outcomes.* Online. Available at: **www.england.nhs.uk/ nursingvision/actions/area-1/** [accessed 31 May 2013].

Ni Shuinear, S. (1997) Why Do Gaujos Hate Gypsies So Much Anyway? A Case Study. In: Acton, T. (Ed.). *Gypsy Politics and Traveller Identity.* Hatfield: University of Hertfordshire Press.

Niner, P. (2003) *Local Authority Gypsy/Traveller Sites in England.* London: ODPM.

Nussbaum, M. and Sen, A. (2006) *The Quality of Life.* Oxford: Clarendon Press.

O'Dowd, A. (2013) Some Health and Wellbeing Boards are too "Pink and Fluffy" and Lack Spine, Expert Warns. *British Medical Journal,* 346, f136.

Offenhauer, P. (2005) *Women in Islamic Society: A Selected Review of the Social Scientific Literature.* Washington DC: Federal Research Division, The Library of Congress.

Office for National Statistics (2012) *Guide to Social Capital.* Online. Available at: **www. ons.gov.uk/ons/guide-method/user-guidance/social-capital-guide/the-social-capital- project/guide-to-social-capital.html** [accessed 15 January 2012].

Office for National Statistics (2013) *Statistical Bulletin: Life Expectancy at Birth and at Age 65 for Local Areas in England and Wales, 2009–11.* Online. Available at: **www.ons.gov.uk/ ons/rel/subnational-health4/life-expectancy-at-birth-and-at-age-65-by-local-areas- in-england-and-wales/2009-11/stb.html** [accessed 9 August 2013].

Office for National Statistics (2014) *Topic Guide to Older People.* Online. Available at: **www. statistics.gov.uk/hub/population/ageing/older-people** [accessed 1 December 2013].

Okely, J. (1983) *The Traveller Gypsies.* Cambridge: University of Cambridge Press.

Parliamentary Office of Science and Technology (2011) *Housing and Health Post Note,* number 371. Online. Available at: **www.parliament.uk/documents/post/postpn_371- housing_health_h.pdf** [accessed 11 September 2013].

Parry, G., Van Cleemput, P., Peters, J., Moore, J., Walters, S., Thomas, K. and Cooper, C. (2004) *The Health Status of Gypsies and Travellers in England.* Sheffield: The University of Sheffield.

Peate, I. (2012) Cherry Picking: Health and Wellbeing Boards. *British Journal of Nursing,* 21(21), 1249.

Peel, N. M., Travers, C., Bell, R. A. R. and Smith, K. (2010) Evaluation of a Health Service Delivery Intervention to Promote Falls Prevention in Older People Across the Care Continuum. *Journal of Evaluation in Clinical Practice,* 16, 1254–1261.

Peters, M. and Marshall, J. (1996) *Individualism and Community: Education and Social Policy in the Postmodern Condition.* London: Falmer Press.

Pitts, M. (1996) *The Psychology of Preventative Health*. London: Routledge.

Portas, M. (2011) *The Portas Review: An Independent Review into the Future of our High Streets*. Online. Available at: **www.bis.gov.uk/assets/BISCore/business-sectors/docs/p/11-1434-portas-review-future-of-high-streets.pdf** [accessed 17 July 2013].

Powell, C. (2008) Understanding the Stigmatization of Gypsies: Power and the Dialectics of (Dis)identification. *Housing, Theory and Society*, 25(2), 87–109.

Powell, J. L. and Hendricks, J. (2009) The Sociological Construction of Ageing: Lessons for Theorising. *International Journal of Sociology and Social Policy*, 29(1/2), 84–94.

Power, C. (2003) Irish Travellers, Ethnicity, Racism and Pre-Sentence Reports. *Probation Journal*, 50(3), 252–266.

Pro-Housing Alliance (2012) *Poor Homes, Poor Health – to Heat or to Eat? Private Sector Tenant Choices in 2012: An Exploratory Study of the Health Impacts of Welfare Reform on Tenants Living in the Private Rented Sector*. Online. Available at: **www.prohousingalliance.com/wp-content/uploads/2012/11/GLHS-report-final4-11-12W2007NoLogo.pdf** [accessed 28 June 2013].

Pulse (2011) *Health and Wellbeing Boards to Determine 'Success or Failure' of Local Commissioning*. Online. Available at: **www.pulsetoday.co.uk/health-and-wellbeing-boards-to-determine-success-or-failure-of-local-commissioning/12269152.article#.UgVZ46w1noo** [accessed 9 August 2013].

Putnam, H. (2006) Objectivity and the Science–Ethics Distinction. In: Nussbaum, M. and Sen, A. (Eds) *The Quality of Life*. Oxford: Clarendon Press.

Quadir, M. (2005) *Discover Islam: The Muslim Woman*. Virginia, USA.

Quadir, M. (2006) *Discover Islam: The Reader*. Virginia, USA.

Quran, The Holy: Arabic Text and English Translation (2004) Surrey: Islamic International Publications.

Ramage, M. and Shipp, K. (2009) *Systems Thinkers*. London: Springer.

Richardson, J. and O'Neill, R. (2012) "Stamp on the Camps": The Social Construction of Gypsies and Travellers in Media and Political Debate. In: Richardson, J. and Ryder, A. (Eds) *Gypsies and Travellers: Empowerment and Inclusion in British Society*. Bristol: Policy Press.

Rittel, H. and Webber, M. (1973) Dilemmas in a General Theory of Planning. *Policy Sciences*, 4(2), 155–169.

Sachs, J. (2013) Restoring Virtue Ethics in the Quest for Happiness. In: Helliwell, J., Layard, R. and Sachs, J. (Eds) *World Happiness Report*. New York: Earth Institute, Columbia University.

Saunders, R. (2012) Crisis? What Crisis? Thatcherism and the Seventies. In: Jackson, B. and Saunders, R. (Eds) *Making Thatcher's Britain*. Cambridge: Cambridge University Press.

Scott, J. C. (1985) *Weapons of the Weak: Everyday Forms of Peasant Resistance*. New Haven: Yale University Press.

Scott-Samuel, A. (2011) *The New Public Health Landscape – Will it Deliver a More Equal Society?* Paper presented at the 'A Climate for Health' Conference, West Bromwich: UK.

Sedlacek, T. (2011) *Economics of Good and Evil: The Quest for Economic Meaning from Gilgamesh to Wall Street*. Oxford: Oxford University Press.

Shahran, M. F. M. (2009) Happiness in Islam. Online. Available at: **http://farshah-ibanah. blogspot.com/2009/11/happiness-in-islam.html** [accessed 30 November 2013].

Sillett, J. (2012) Health and Social Care Bill: Health and Wellbeing Boards. *British Journal of Nursing*, 21(12), 710.

Smelser, N. (2004) Psychological and Cultural Trauma. In: Alexander, J.C. *et al*. (Eds) *Cultural Trauma and Collective Identity*. Berkeley, CA: University of California Press.

Smith, A., Humphreys, S., Heslington, L., La Placa, V., McVey, D. and MacGregor, E. (2011) *The Healthy Foundations Lifestage Segmentation, Research Report no. 2: The Qualitative Analysis of the Motivational Segments*. London: Department of Health/National Social Marketing Centre. Online. Available at: **http://thensmc.com/sites/default/files/ HFLS%20Report%20No2_ACC.pdf** [accessed 20 April 2013].

Smith, D. and Greenfields, M. (2012) Housed Gypsies and Travellers in the UK: Work, Exclusion and Adaptation. *Race and Class*, 53(3), 48–65.

Smith, D. and Greenfields, M. (2013) *Gypsies and Travellers in Housing: The Decline of Nomadism*. Bristol: Policy Press.

Smith, K. E., Bambara, C., Joyce, K. E., Perkins, N., Hunter, D. J. and Blenkinsopp, E. A. (2009) Partners in Health? A Systematic Review of the Impact of Organizational Partnerships on Public Health Outcomes in England Between 1997 and 2008. *Journal of Public Health*, 31(2), 210–221.

Social Care Institute for Excellence (2010) *At a Glance 30: Personalisation Briefing - Implications for NHS Staff*. Online. Available at: **www.scie.org.uk/publications/ataglance/ ataglance30.asp** [accessed 1 December 2013].

Social Care Workforce Research Unit (2005) *Update for SCIE Best Practice Guide on Assessing the Mental Health Needs of Older People*. Online. Available at: **www.scie.org.uk/ publications/guides/guide03/framework/wellbeing.asp** [accessed 29 May 2013].

Spear, S., Stewart, J., Knight, A. and Stacey, C. (2011) Wellbeing and Mental Health: An Evolving Role for Environmental Health Practitioners through Evidence Based Practice. *Journal of Environmental Health Research*, 11(3), 117–126.

Spigner, C. and Moreno-Leguizamon, C. (2011) Public Health, Wellbeing and Culture: A Critical Perspective. In: Knight, A. and McNaught, A. (Eds) *Understanding Wellbeing: An Introduction for Students and Practitioners of Health and Social Care*. Banbury: Lantern Publishing.

Staite, C. and Miller, R. (2011) *Health and Wellbeing Boards: Developing a Successful Partnership*. Institute of Local Government Studies Health Services Management Centre. Birmingham: University of Birmingham.

Stedman Jones, D. (2012) *Masters of the Universe: Hayek, Friedman, and the Birth of Neoliberal Politics*. New Jersey: Princeton University Press.

Steiner, L., Leinart, L. and Frey, B. (2010) Economics, Religion and Happiness. *ZFWU – Zeitschrift für Wirtschafts- und Unternehmensethik*, 11(1), 1–17.

Stewart, J. (2013) *Effective Strategies and Interventions: Environmental Health and the Private Housing Sector*. London: Chartered Institute of Environmental Health.

Stewart, J. and Knight, A. (2011) Private Sector Housing Conditions: Influencing Health and Wellbeing Across the Generations. *Perspectives in Public Health*, 131(6), 255–256.

Stewart, J., Bushell, F. and Habgood, V. (2005) *Environmental Health as Public Health*. London: Chadwick House Group.

Stoecker, R. (2013) *Research Methods for Community Change: A Project Based Approach* (2nd edn). London: Sage.

Stonewall. (2003) *Profiles of Prejudice*. London: Stonewall.

Struyk, R. J. and Haddaway, S. R. (2012) Mentoring Policy Research Organisations: Project Evaluation Results. *International Society for Third-Sector Research*, 23, 636–660.

Suleiman, Y. (2013) *Narratives of Conversion to Islam in Britain: Female Perspectives*. Cambridge: Centre for Islamic Studies.

Surr, C., Boyle, G. Brooker, G., Godfrey, M. and Townsend, J. (2005) *Prevention and Service Provision: Mental Health Problems in Later Life*. Leeds: Centre for Health and Social Care.

Sutherland, A. (1975) *Gypsies: The Hidden Americans*. Illinois: Wavelength Press.

Sztompka, P. (2004) The Trauma of Social Change. In: Alexander, J.C. *et al.* (Eds) *Cultural Trauma and Collective Identity*. Berkeley, CA: University of California Press.

Tatz, C. (2004) Aboriginal, Maori and Inuit Youth Suicide: Avenues to Alleviation? *Australian Aboriginal Studies*, 2, 15–25.

Taylor, C. (1989) Overcoming Epistemology. In: Baynes, K. K. J., Bohman, J. and McCarthy, T. (Eds) *Philosophy: End or Transformation?* Cambridge, MA: MIT Press.

Tester, S., Hubbard, G., Downs, M., MacDonald, C. and Murphy, J. (2004) Frailty and Institutional Life. In: Walker, A. and Hagen Hennessey, C. (Eds) *Growing Older: Quality of Life in Old Age.* Maidenhead: Open University Press.

Thanet District Council (2011) *Margate Task Force.* Online. Available at **www.thanet.gov. uk/news/latest_press_releases/margate_task_force_launch.aspx** [accessed 17 December 2011].

The Association of Directors of Children's Services, The Department of Health, The Local Government Group, The NHS Alliance, The NHS Confederation, The Royal College of General Practitioners, The Royal Society for Public Health, Solace (2011) *Operating Principles for Health and Wellbeing Boards: Laying the Foundations for Healthier Places.* London: The NHS Confederation.

The Silver Line (2013) *The Silver Line Helpline for Older People.* Online. Available at: **www. thesilverline.org.uk/** [accessed 13 October 2013].

Thin, N. (2009) Why Anthropology Can Ill Afford to Ignore Well-Being. In: Mathews, G. and Izquierdo, C. (Eds) *Pursuits of Happiness: Well-Being in Anthropological Perspective.* New York: Berghahn Books.

Thomas, P. A. and Campbell, S. (1992) *Housing Gypsies.* Cardiff: Traveller Law Research Unit.

Tiliouine, H., Cummins, R. A. and Davern, M. (2009) Islamic Religiosity, Subjective Wellbeing and Health. *Mental Health, Religion and Culture,* 12(1), 55–74.

Tomlinson, J. (1991) *Cultural Imperialism: A Critical Introduction.* Baltimore: The Johns Hopkins University Press.

Townsend, P., Davidson, N. and Whitehead, M. (1988) *Inequalities in Health: The Black Report and The Health Divide.* Harmondsworth: Penguin.

Tovar-Restrepo, M. (2012) *Castoriadis, Foucault, and Autonomy: New Approaches to Subjectivity, Society and Social Change.* London: Bloomsbury.

Tranel, M. and Handlin, L. B. (2006) Metromorphosis: Documenting Change. *Journal of Urban Affairs,* 28, 151–167.

Turner, R. J. (1981) Social Support as a Contingency in Psychological Well-Being. *Journal of Health and Social Behaviour,* 22(4), 357–367.

Turner, E., Henryks, J. and Pearson, D. (2010) *Community Garden Conference: Promoting Sustainability, Health and Inclusion in the City.* Online. Available at: **www.canberra.edu.au/ communitygardens/home** [accessed 30 September 2013].

Turner, D., Salway, S., Mir, G., Ellison, G. T., Skinner, J., Carter, L. and Bostan, B. (2013) Prospects for Progress on Health Inequalities in England in the Post-Primary Care Trust Era: Professional Views on Challenges, Risks and Opportunities. *BioMedCentral Public Health*, 13, 274.

U3A (2013) Life is for Learning. Online. Available at: **www.u3a.org.uk/** [accessed 13 October 2013].

United Nations Development Programme (2013) *Human Development Report: The Rise of the South: Human Progress in a Diverse World*. New York: United Nations Development Programme.

Voicu, I. and Been, V. (2008) The Effect of Community Gardens on Neighboring Property Values. *Real Estate Economics*, 36(2), 241–283.

Walker, P. and Longley, M. (2012) A Greatest Wellbeing Principle: Its Time has Come. In: Walker, P. and John, M. (Eds) *From Public Health to Wellbeing: The New Driver for Policy and Action*. London: Palgrave.

Walton, J. and Browne, P. (2010) *Coastal Regeneration in English Resorts*. Lincoln: Coastal Communities Alliance.

Wan Ibrahim, W. A., Zainab, I., Asyraf, H. A. R. and Fadzil, A. (2012) Subjective Wellbeing of Older Rural Muslim Community in Malaysia. *International Journal of Asian Social Science*, 2(3), 330–335.

Weller, P., Feldman, A. and Purdam, K. (2001) *Religious Discrimination in England and Wales, Home Office Research Study 220*. London: Home Office.

Whitmore, E., Guijt, I., Mertons, D. M., Imm, P. S., Chinman, M. and Wandersman, A. (2013) Embedding Improvements, Lived Experiences, and Social Justice in Evaluation Practice. In: Shaw, I., Greene, J. and Mark, M. (Eds) *The Sage Handbook of Evaluation*. London: Sage.

Whitney, W., Dutcher, G. A. and Keselman, A. (2009) Evaluation of Health Information Outreach: Theory, Practice and Future Direction. *Journal of the Medical Library Association*, 101(2), 138–146.

Wilkinson, R. and Pickett, K. (2010). *The Spirit Level: Why Equality is Better for Everyone*. London: Penguin.

Willers, M. (2010) *Facilitating the Gypsy and Traveller Way of Life in England and Wales through the Courts*. Paper presented at 'Romani Mobilities in Europe' Conference: Oxford.

Willetts, D. (2010) *The Pinch: How the Baby Boomers Took Their Children's Future – And Why They Should Give It Back*. London: Atlantic Books.

Williams, B., McVey, D., Davies, L. and MacGregor, E. (2011) *The Healthy Foundations Lifestages Segmentation, Research Report no. 1: Creating the Segmentation Using a Quantitative Survey of the General Population of England*. London: Department of Health/National Social Marketing Centre. Online. Available at: **http://thensmc.com/sites/default/files/301846_HFLS%20Report%20No1_ACC.pdf** [accessed 26 May 2013].

Willis Commission (2012) *Quality with Compassion: The Future of Nursing Education*. Online. Available at: **www.williscommission.org.uk/__data/assets/pdf_file/0007/495115/Willis_commission_report_Jan_2013.pdf** [accessed 26 May 2013].

Wilson, O. and Hughes, O. (2011) Urban Green Space Policy and Discourse in England under New Labour from 1997 to 2010. *Planning Practice and Research*, 26(2), 207–228.

Wood, C., Ragg, R., Pretty, J. and Barton, J. (2012) *The Health Benefits of the "Generations Growing Together" (GGT Community Allotments Project). Short Report for Essex County Council*. University of Essex. Online. Available at: **www.greenexercise.org/pdf/GGT%20main%20report.pdf** [accessed 30 September 2013].

Woodlock, R. (2012) Muslim Wellbeing in Australia: Analysis of Personal and National Wellbeing among a Sample of Muslims Living in NSW and Victoria. *Islam and Christian Relations*, 23, 181–200.

World Health Organization (1946) *Constitution*. Geneva: WHO.

World Health Organization (2013) *Definition of an Older Person or Elderly Person*. Online. Available at: **www.who.int/healthinfo/survey/ageingdefnolder/en/** [accessed 26 May 2013].

World Health Organization and Commission on the Social Determinants of Health. (2008) *Closing the Gap in a Generation: Health Equity Through Action on the Social Determinants of Health*. Online. Available at: **http://whqlibdoc.who.int/publications/2008/9789241563703_eng.pdf** [accessed 11 September 2013].

Wynne-Jones, R. (2013) *Deserving vs Undeserving*. Online. Available at: **www.jrf.org.uk/reporting-poverty/journalists-experiences/deserving-undeserving** [accessed 9 August 2013].

INDEX